ADDICTION AND ART

Addiction and Art

Patricia B. Santora
The Johns Hopkins University School of Medicine
Baltimore, Maryland

Margaret L. Dowell
Mount St. Mary's University
Emmitsburg, Maryland, and
Carroll Community College
Westminster, Maryland

Jack E. Henningfield
The Johns Hopkins University School of Medicine
Baltimore, Maryland, and
Pinney Associates
Bethesda, Maryland

THE JOHNS HOPKINS UNIVERSITY PRESS
Baltimore

© 2010 The Johns Hopkins University Press
All rights reserved. Published 2010
Printed in Canada on acid-free paper
9 8 7 6 5 4 3 2 1

The Johns Hopkins University Press
2715 North Charles Street
Baltimore, Maryland 21218-4363

www.press.jhu.edu

Library of Congress Cataloging-in-Publication Data

Addiction and art / edited by Patricia B. Santora, Margaret L. Dowell, Jack E.
Henningfield.
       p. ; cm.
    Includes bibliographical references.
    ISBN-13: 978-0-8018-9481-7 (hardcover : alk. paper)
    ISBN-10: 0-8018-9481-6 (hardcover : alk. paper)
    1. Drug addiction. 2. Art. I. Santora, Patricia B., 1949– II. Dowell, Margaret L.
III. Henningfield, Jack E.
    [DNLM: 1. Substance-Related Disorders—psychology. 2. Art Therapy. 3. Medicine in
Art. 4. Substance-Related Disorders—rehabilitation. WM 270 A22309 2010]
    HV5801.A275 2010
    362.29022'2—dc22   2009030922

A catalog record for this book is available from the British Library.

*Special discounts are available for bulk purchases of this book. For more information, please
contact Special Sales at 410-516-6936 or specialsales@press.jhu.edu.*

The Johns Hopkins University Press uses environmentally friendly book materials,
including recycled text paper that is composed of at least 30 percent post-consumer waste,
whenever possible. All of our book papers are acid-free, and our jackets and covers are
printed on paper with recycled content.

It is art that *makes* life, makes interest, makes importance…
and I know of no substitute whatever for the force and beauty of its
process.

Henry James to H. G. Wells
Letter of July 10, 1915
21 Carlyle Mansions, Cheyne Walk, London

CONTENTS

ACKNOWLEDGMENTS

We gratefully acknowledge the grant support of the Robert Wood Johnson Foundation, whose sponsorship through the Innovators Combating Substance Abuse Awards Program made this unique book possible. Early encouragement of the concept of art as a viable and important approach for communication as well as a complement to science in understanding the human side of addiction was provided by former Surgeon General C. Everett Koop, American Visionary Art Museum's founder and director, Rebecca Alban Hoffberger, former first lady of Maryland Kendel Ehrlich, and Innovator Award recipient Ray Materson.

We are indebted to the members of the Innovators' Addiction Art Advisory Board (see Appendix A), who committed two days to a "think tank" meeting to review and select the art and to discuss the pivotal role that addiction art plays in education about, treatment of, and prevention of substance use disorders.

We are grateful to Keith Weller of Columbia, Maryland, for his superb photography of the original art contained in this book. Mr. Weller photographed the majority of the art while it was on display at the annual meeting of the College on Problems of Drug Dependence, San Juan, Puerto Rico, June 2008.

We appreciate the excellent editorial assistance of the editors and staff of the Johns Hopkins University Press in preparing this book.

Most of all, we are grateful to the contributing artists whose art highlights the need to seek more effective ways to treat addictions and to help individuals achieve recovery.

INTRODUCTION

This book marks the intersection of science and the visual arts. It captures the real-world experience of addiction and recovery as revealed through the visual arts and the written word. Organizing a collection of art devoted to substance abuse and addiction could be seen as falling outside the sphere of addiction science. What does art have to do with addiction, anyway? Science helps to explain the phenomena of addiction, but artistic expression helps us to understand it in a way that is complementary and no less insightful. Science gives us the tools, but art gives us the inspiration and the drive to make a difference in reducing addiction and helping people achieve recovery. What is more important—the tools or the drive? They are inseparable.

By combining science with art, two seemingly disparate disciplines, we seek not to supplant the scientific view of addiction and its treatment but to complement it. Our primary goal for this collection of art is to reveal the human experience of addiction so that readers may reach a new understanding of addiction as a chronic medical illness requiring treatment. With this view of addiction directing our efforts, we adopted the fundamental strategy that former Surgeon General C. Everett Koop proposed: to fight addiction instead of fighting those who have it.

Addiction science tells us that substance abuse and addiction are among the most prevalent, deadly, and costly health problems in the United States. They account for approximately one in five deaths annually—500,000 persons—and more than one-half trillion U.S. dollars. With the medical, social, and psychological toll from undiagnosed and untreated substance abuse reaching epidemic status, what can be done to refocus our country's strategies to prevent and reduce the harm caused by substance abuse?

Addiction art conveys the human experience of addiction that lies hidden behind the statistics of addiction science. It shows us how individuals, families, and communities live with addiction. Addiction art reveals the many-faceted struggles of those entrapped in a life ruled by addiction. Whereas science analyzes and explains addiction using data displayed in pie charts and bar graphs, art reveals the tangled complexity of addiction through works made of paint and other materials to enhance our understanding of this treatable chronic illness.

Our intent is to help people from all walks of life recognize, first and foremost, that addiction is never only about alcoholics or addicts; it is also about the families and communities whose lives intertwine with those of addicted persons in myriad ways. We hope these art works, individually and collectively, will make it easier for all of us to welcome people with addictions back into the human community.

This volume provides opportunities to raise consciousness and change behavior. By engaging people's feelings and perceptions, art can help change awareness. We hope that these images will highlight the need to continue seeking more effective ways to treat addictions and thereby help individuals achieve recovery and become integrated into the everyday lives of our communities in positive ways. We also hope that the collection highlights the importance of prevention and re-energizes efforts to reach out to individuals at risk, especially young people.

This collection represents an extraordinary collaboration among individuals from very different communities: the artists whose work is represented here and a unique advisory group of addiction scientists and art professionals. The contributing artists brought their individual talents and experience with the world of addiction to the works they submitted. The members of our advisory group brought not only their professional expertise to the endeavor but also their personal experience of art. Many also brought a perspective influenced by close personal contact with a family member, friend, or colleague suffering from substance abuse or addiction.

We envision this volume to appeal to a diverse audience: the general public, individuals in recovery, health professionals working within and outside of addiction medicine, young people, community leaders, and policymakers. Through these images, we hope readers will better understand the experience of addiction and, in the process, reclaim a human connection with individuals who suffer from this treatable chronic illness.

For two prospective audiences in particular—individuals in recovery and young people—our advisory group questioned whether some images in this volume would be inappropriate. Did images contain triggers that might provoke relapse or promote experimentation? They were particularly concerned about the seductive quality of some images with respect to young audiences. Of equal concern was whether parents, educators, community leaders, or others might find some images inappropriate for young people— for example, images that involved nudity or grotesque representations of the body as well as images that glamorized drug use. Would including such images lead to the collection's being barred from use in schools, churches, or community youth programs?

Our advisory group discussed these concerns repeatedly, as they were raised in one form or another by different pieces. They struggled not only with the needs and sensibilities of our potential audiences but also with a somewhat disturbing question of self-censorship. Ultimately, it was difficult, if not impossible, to predict what would offend readers. An image that one individual finds objectionable, another may find deeply moving. We recognized that, by its very nature and subject matter, this collection of art would be challenging, no matter which works were selected.

It is vital to reach young people and young adults. Research has shown that addiction begins much earlier than once thought.[1] Audiences of high school age and even younger need to understand addiction if they are to avoid it. Especially important is reaching America's college students, since the prevailing college culture of binge drinking—engaged in by as many as one-half of full-time college students[2]—threatens the stability and future of our country. Solutions are urgently needed to stop the best and the brightest at America's colleges and universities from wasting their lives because of binge drinking.

To reach young audiences, this collection of art needed to be forthright. Honest images of addiction are necessarily also troubling images, whether because they allude to pleasurable facets of addictive behaviors or because they are brutal in their depiction of the consequences of such behavior. In producing this volume, we discussed several strategies for balancing the need to address the sensibilities of prospective audiences, the need to maintain the artistic and intellectual honesty of the collection, and our overarching goal of using the collection as a tool to humanize the experience of addiction and recovery.

The book consists of three sections. Chapter 1 describes the rationale for cultivating the visual arts to stimulate insights into addiction and recovery. It presents key facts about substance abuse and addiction, discusses the current state of addiction treatment, and describes how addiction scientists are using addiction science to improve treatment and build better systems of care.

Essential to this chapter is a discussion of how to change the way Americans view addiction by using the visual arts to reveal the human face of addiction and recovery. The underlying goal of this volume is for the visual arts to complement addiction science.

Chapter 2 discusses how the visual arts tell the complex story of addiction and recovery. Descriptions are provided of juried Art and Addiction exhibitions and how they have enriched addiction science presentations at professional conferences. Particularly important in this chapter is a description of the guidelines and process used to judge and select the art contained in this volume. Chapter 3, the book's centerpiece, presents the art together with the artists' brief statements about their work, documenting stories of addiction and recovery. The epilogue discusses several key consensus points that underscore the pivotal role that addiction art plays in the education about and prevention of substance use disorders.

We hope this collection will be engaging and stimulate thinking about addiction in a new light—as a chronic medical illness requiring treatment. More prosaically, we intend this collection to illustrate the value of art as a tool for health communications by educators and advocates. We envision it being used to introduce addiction studies, as an easy and effective way to engage students entering the field of addiction medicine or community groups and policymakers grappling with how to address the complexities of addiction and create paths to recovery.

ADDICTION AND ART

ONE

Cultivating the Visual Arts to Stimulate Insights into Addiction and Recovery

Substance abuse and addiction to alcohol, tobacco, and illicit and/or prescription drugs are leading public health problems of our time. Substance abuse/addiction is a major contributor to heart disease, cancer, and stroke, the three main causes of death in the United States.[1] Our hospitals are filled with patients whose illnesses are severely complicated by substance abuse/addiction.[2] Patients diagnosed with medical illnesses who also have substance use disorders do not follow prescribed medical care and have poorer treatment outcomes, more hospitalizations, and increased costs.[3] With 435,000 deaths annually from tobacco, 85,000 deaths from alcohol, and 17,000 deaths from illicit drug use, substance abuse/addiction accounts for 1 of every 5 deaths in the United States.[4]

The economic impact of substance abuse/addiction is enormous. The combined costs of health care and lost productivity are estimated at more than one-half trillion U.S. dollars—approximately $170 billion for tobacco dependence,[5] $180 billion for alcohol abuse and dependence,[6] and $185 billion for illicit drug abuse.[7] Given the immense health and economic burdens it inflicts, substance abuse/addiction has reached epidemic status; it is one of our most urgent public health problems, requiring vigorous and immediate action.

Compared to other medical illnesses, however, substance abuse/addiction receives little attention from the medical and public health communities. The reasons for this are many, ranging from the perception that substance abuse is primarily a social problem requiring law enforcement intervention, not a health problem requiring treatment, to skepticism about the efficacy of addiction treatment, as well as poorly funded research, weak leadership, stigma, and stereotypes.[8] Many of these obstacles to appropriate action, however, are caused more by indifference and prejudice.

Substance abuse/addiction is a complex medical, public health, and social problem. Reducing the harm caused by substance use disorders presents formidable challenges. As a nation, can we develop useful strategies that will prevent and reduce substance abuse/addiction as was done for other public health challenges such as polio, tuberculosis, and HIV/AIDS?

Former Surgeon General C. Everett Koop, in a recent editorial on improving our nation's health and health care in the twenty-first century, highlighted addiction treatment as an area of unrealized potential and called on public health professionals to chart a new course.[9] He observed that "the solution to drug addiction won't come until it is as easy to find treatment for drug addiction as it is to find addictive drugs."[10]

The Current State of Addiction Treatment

Addiction treatment must be readily available, but, like the lives of many addicted individuals, the state of addiction treatment in the United States is in disarray.[11] Major gaps exist between what research has shown to be effective addiction treatment and what is practiced in clinical settings.[12] Furthermore, leading addiction scientists have reached an "unsettling consensus" that our society has no organized system of care to meet the treatment needs of those with substance abuse/addiction.[13] To summarize, current research shows that addiction treatment:

- is not readily available for those who need it;[14]
- is not integrated into mainstream medicine[15] but remains segregated in programs offering treatments that are not science-driven;[16] and
- is forever vulnerable to pendulum shifts in funding priorities from one health risk to another (e.g., treating nicotine addiction versus child-hood obesity).[17]

Addiction scientists are addressing these shortcomings, using excellent addiction science to improve treatment. Furthermore, the Institute of Medicine recently issued specific recommendations for addressing the unmet health care needs of those with substance abuse/addiction who also have co-occurring medical and psychiatric disorders.[18] In addition to improving treatment, addiction scientists are also striving to build better systems of care based on a coherent set of much-needed guidelines for the field.[19]

Reviewing the health and economic burdens of substance abuse/addiction is the standard approach of addiction science. But a scientific perspective alone can never offer a complete portrayal of substance abuse/addiction. Addiction science does not capture the suffering of individuals entrapped in a life ruled by substance abuse/addiction, nor does it depict the distress of families watching in anguish while a loved one struggles with this medical illness.

Changing the Way Americans View Addiction

Preventing and reducing substance abuse/addiction rests not only on changing how addiction is treated but also on changing the way Americans view addiction—that is, persuading them that addiction is neither a weakness nor a "moral failing" deserving of punishment but, instead, a chronic medical illness requiring treatment. The management of this illness would be similar to the medical management of other chronic illnesses such as hypertension, diabetes, or AIDS. Understanding addiction as a treatable medical illness is essential in preventing this prevalent public health problem. With this view of addiction directing our efforts, we can fight substance abuse/addiction instead of fighting those who have it.

To change misconceptions about substance abuse/addiction, we can offer valuable lessons from HIV/AIDS, the other prominent epidemic of our time. As a nation, we have responded more vigorously over the past 25 years to prevent AIDS and to treat those who have it than we have responded to those who suffer from substance abuse/addiction. Part of the reason for this response was that the HIV/AIDS community used art to portray the human experience of what it meant to suffer from this disease and its devastating consequences. They enlisted artists to tell the AIDS story and to document the impact of the AIDS epidemic through several artistic endeavors, including novels (e.g., *And the Band Played On*),[20] Pulitzer Prize–winning plays (e.g., *Angels in America*),[21] and memoirs (e.g., *Borrowed Time*).[22] Artists charted the course of the AIDS epidemic to place it within the broader context of how disease and society interact.

Perhaps the best known work of art documenting the AIDS epidemic is the AIDS Memorial Quilt, the world's largest community art project. Based on the latest estimate from more than 35 countries, the quilt comprises more than 46,000 individual 3- by 6-foot memorial panels, each honoring one particular person who died of AIDS. Over the past 20 years, the quilt has been seen by more than 15 million people and has raised several millions of dollars for AIDS service organizations.[23] The quilt is a powerful statement, showing compassion for those who were afflicted—compassion that was transformed into passion to help find new ways to treat this fatal disease. Science was called on to provide a path to life, but art gave the reason. Art was one of the many powerful tools that helped build awareness and influence health-related agencies to join together to fight the AIDS epidemic. A unique leadership coalition—consisting of the Centers for Disease Control and Prevention, the National Institutes of Health, the Food and Drug Administration, the pharmaceutical industry, health philanthropies, and advocacy organizations—transformed AIDS, considered a death sentence in the early 1980s, into a treatable chronic disease by the 1990s.

Similar to the AIDS artists who used art to stimulate discussion and to advocate for more treatment and medication development, we can change the way Americans view addiction by using the visual arts to reveal the human face of addiction and recovery. We need the visual arts to help refocus our country's attention on the critical need for addiction treatment, additional research funding, stronger leadership, and effective alcohol, tobacco, and drug policies to prevent and reduce the harm from substance abuse/ addiction.

Visual artists, with or without personal experience with substance abuse, can provide insights into the human features of addiction and recovery. Art can exemplify the human experience of addiction by opening the door to understanding and provoking a compassionate response. As noted by one of the artists in this volume, "It is important to communicate what it is like to be in the grip of addiction. The fear and agony that drive an addiction are prisons that only bring pain and desperation…The road to recovery would be more accessible if it were paved with understanding."

By revealing the human face of addiction, art helps the mainstream community find innovative, positive ways to engage with the world of addiction and recovery. By opening a door to that world, art helps us overcome the temptation to view addiction as "a matter of bad people making bad choices —nothing to do with *us*." Another artist featured in this volume commented on the value of art as "a portal that allows us to see past our own worldly constructs into the unknown." By inviting us to engage with the experience of addiction and recovery in an immediate, personal, and often visceral way, art helps us move beyond stigma and stereotypes to recognize that substance abuse and addiction are *our* problem as a community, not just *their* failing as individuals.

We hold the unwavering belief that creativity and artistic expression can play a significant role in raising awareness of the personal toll caused by substance abuse/addiction and of the new life born in recovery. Our goal is not to supplant the scientific view of addiction but to complement it. Addiction art is the complementary universe to addiction science, providing insights that the science cannot offer and bridging the gap between the science and the human experience of addiction. In treating addiction, art is as necessary as science because, if we do not have the passion to understand and to help, the science may go unused.

TWO

How the Visual Arts Capture the Complexity of Addiction

Drawing on the visual arts to provide insights into addiction and recovery was an integral component of the national program office of Innovators Combating Substance Abuse, which two of the editors (JEH and PBS) co-directed. This program was supported by the Robert Wood Johnson Foundation and was based in the Department of Psychiatry and Behavioral Sciences at the Johns Hopkins University School of Medicine. The goal was to foster innovation in reducing and controlling substance abuse/addiction by granting awards to leading individuals working in the substance abuse field and through the use of strategically planned initiatives.

The Innovators program organized five juried Art and Addiction exhibitions (2004–2008), promoting the use of art to complement science in understanding addiction and recovery. The addiction art exhibitions dealt with legal drugs (alcohol, tobacco, prescription) as well as illegal ones (marijuana, cocaine, heroin, etc.). The art displayed a broad spectrum of artists' perspectives on drug use and abuse, addiction, altered states of consciousness, and recovery from addiction. Through their art, talented visual artists provided valuable insight by capturing both the destructive power of addiction and the new life born in recovery. The stories of drug abuse and addiction, drug problems, and efforts to prevent and treat these problems have been told through a variety of media. The Innovators' addiction art exhibitions have featured paintings, sculptures, needlework, photography, prints, drawings, ceramics, decorative arts, video art, and other artifacts.

The Art and Addiction exhibitions were held in conjunction with national substance abuse conferences for professionals in the field (e.g., the annual meeting of the College on Problems of Drug Dependence as well as the Dr. Lonnie Mitchell National Substance Abuse Conference for Historically Black Colleges and Universities). The art has also been displayed at the central headquarters of our country's Substance Abuse and Mental Health Services Administration in Rockville, Maryland. The exhibitions have been considered an essential component or, as one professional commented, "a perfect match to the ongoing scientific discussions" at professional meetings. The growing consensus among substance abuse professionals confirms that addiction art complements addiction science and is a "remarkable contribution to the field of substance abuse prevention and treatment." As described by one professional in the addictions field, the addiction art exhibition "provides inspiration for our sometimes disheartening work."

With these endorsements, the Innovators program extended its addiction art exhibitions to the next level using the community college network. We collaborated with the leadership of Carroll Community College in Westminster, Maryland, with the goal of educating the broader community about preventing and treating addiction using our model of addiction art exhibitions. We expanded our model to include art created not only by established artists but also by emerging student artists in high school and college. Response to the community college exhibitions on addiction art resulted in a tremendous groundswell of interest from the community, making it the most popular art exhibition in the college's twenty-year history. Unprecedented crowds and constant media interest ignited widespread curiosity, and diverse community groups of all ages visited the campus daily to see the artwork during the six-week exhibition period.

Several pieces of addiction art from these exhibitions were published in our recent book on addiction treatment,[1] where addiction art was prominently displayed with essays on addiction science. The art published in that book was compelling to the Johns Hopkins University Press, and it provided the basis to undertake this separate volume devoted exclusively to art and addiction.

The art featured in this book was selected by the Innovators' Addiction Art Advisory Board, a unique group of addiction scientists and art professionals (professors, curators, and gallery owners). A complete list of advisory board members is provided in Appendix A. In response to a national "Call to Artists" that was widely circulated through print and electronic media, the advisory group reviewed approximately 1,000 art submissions from 394 artists who reside in 42 states, the District of Columbia, and Puerto Rico. Submissions were also received from artists in 13 foreign countries. Specific details about methods used in collecting the art for this book are given in Appendix B.

Addiction Art Selections

In organizing the art for this volume, we focused on one key question: Should the images be selected because they are considered good or strong works of art or because they convey powerful messages about addiction?

One possible answer was to select "outstanding art," where the focus would be on the individual merits of each piece as a work of art in and of itself. Advisory members from the art community were helping the group as a whole to appreciate technical matters, such as composition and use of media. Given our hopes for the collection, could we afford to include art for art's sake—even a piece that challenged a viewer to discern its message?

Another possible answer was to select art that offered a compelling message about addiction regardless of technical sophistication or degree of artistic sensibility. Using that criterion we would focus on the story that a piece conveyed. If a submission carried a unique message, we wondered, how much should it matter that it might be less accomplished or less worthy of praise as a work of art than other pieces under consideration?

The advisory group agreed that, although they were committed to choosing artworks of high quality, they would include pieces that carried a message about addiction which would contribute to our broader goals for the volume. For the collection to succeed, it needed to speak to a wide audience while also winning credibility in the art and scientific communities.

In addition to submitting a photograph of their submission, artists were invited to include a brief written statement about their art. Consequently, along with the broad question of artistry versus message, the advisory group also considered a second recurring question: how to balance the weight given to the piece relative to the artist's statement—an image-versus-text discussion. If our goal was to tell a story, did we expect the art alone to tell it, or did we see the story as emerging from a synergy of the image and statement? Should we consider the pieces as freestanding works or as illustrations that would accompany the text?

To a certain extent, our responses broke along "party lines": members of the art community on the panel maintained that the image should dominate, with commentary playing a supporting role. Members of the addiction medicine community were often less certain that images alone could truly tell the addiction story effectively for a wide audience. We concluded that the collection would be most effective if conceived and presented as multilayered, encompassing both the image and the artist's voice in his or her statement.

A related issue concerned what balance to strike among different types of images in the collection overall. Some of the images are very literal; *Ticket to Recovery*, for example, uses text *as* the image very effectively. Others, like *Blood Bubbles*, are abstract; while still others exemplify "outsider art" (e.g., *Get Humble Now*). There are pieces of narrative art, rich in visual cues, telling the addiction story (*Toy Soldier*); there are still lifes (*Three Square*) and pieces in a folk art style (*My Pill Girl*). Some works are wrenching; some are humorous. We recognized the need to include images with positive valences, and we also sought to balance narrative and expressive art with works more abstract and understated.

We wanted the collection as a whole to address all aspects of addiction, from its allure and destructiveness to the new life found in treatment and recovery. We also wanted the collection to include all modes of addiction, from the use of legal drugs (alcohol and tobacco) and illegal drugs to the abuse of prescription drugs as well as other addictive behaviors such as eating and gambling disorders. It was important for the images to underscore that addiction is an equal opportunity affliction; it does not discriminate on the basis of gender, age, family background, or financial status. Women and children are as susceptible as men; no ethnic or cultural group or community is immune; the poor and the well-to-do are equally vulnerable.

Above all else, we recognized that the selected images had to be accessible. We were keenly aware of how important it is that readers not feel intimidated. Individual works could be disturbing; some might be repulsive. As one of our advisors remarked, "Some pieces you like; others you remember." They might seduce or frighten, elicit sorrow or anger, but they must not leave readers feeling that they cannot understand, on some level, what is at stake.

Telling Stories

With these guidelines directing our efforts, we explored our responses to individual works and identified reasons for selecting them for this collection. Advisory members discussed the stories revealed by the works. Art professionals enriched the conversation by discussing how the pieces conveyed their meanings and stories. Addiction practitioners and researchers noted how some works highlighted key scientific facets of addiction and recovery. Both groups appreciated the social and cultural implications revealed through the art.

This collection tells many diverse stories about addiction—stories of pain and confusion (*Living Hell*), despair (*Fast Exit*), grief (*River of Tears, Matthew, Goodbye, Drowning*), numbness, and isolation, alongside stories of hope (*Restoration of the Spirit*), love, comfort, and connection (*Prodigal Son*). Some pieces tell stories about how addiction captures the mind (*My Pill Girl*) and how it ravages the body (*Boils*). They teach us to remember that addicted individuals are always aware of their addiction and that they know what they are losing even as they continue their addictive behavior (*I'm Dying for a Smoke*; *Now that You're Gone I Can't Apologize*). Many of these images reinforce how terribly hard it is to quit (*My Kingdom for a Horse*) and not relapse (*Recovery*). Some of the works tell stories about the pleasure, beauty, and seductiveness that lie behind addictions (*Number 11*). Those stories are especially disturbing, speaking to something many feel is better left unknown. And yet, these stories are honest, and if addiction is to be addressed effectively, we must in turn be honest in recognizing and understanding them.

Our advisory group did not always read the same story in an art piece. From a single work, one group member might read the story of an addicted person's profound loss of hope while another took from it a story of recovery and yet another, a story about what life is like for someone who loves / hates / grieves for an addicted person. The most powerful pieces are multi-layered, multi-vocal, and textured in extraordinary and sometimes quite unexpected ways (*Toy Soldier, Prodigal Son, The Annunciation*).

As each artwork told its story—or stories —our advisory group appreciated more fully how vividly the collection as a whole captured the complexity of addiction. This collection embodies one master story: addiction and recovery are not and have never been simple phenomena. They do, however, involve human individuals who, in the most fundamental ways, are no different from those of us who have not been addicted. As a member of our advisory group, former Surgeon General C. Everett Koop, summed up one of the most prominent messages conveyed in this collection: no matter how badly entangled in addiction an individual may be, "we *must* treat every addicted person as recoverable."

THREE

Art Complements Science
A Collection of Addiction Art and Artists' Statements

The addiction art in this chapter is a stunning collection documenting the stories of individuals struggling and recovering from addiction. The art has been created by artists recovering from addiction and also by non-addicted artists who have shown through their art how addiction destroys individuals, families, and communities. This collection of 61 artworks created by 57 artists features all drugs of abuse—including the legal drugs of alcohol and tobacco, illegal drugs (for example, marijuana, heroin, cocaine), and prescription drugs—and also examines other behavioral conditions such as eating and gambling disorders. The art displays a broad spectrum of artists' perspectives on drug use and abuse, addiction, and recovery. These stories are told through a variety of media: paintings, sculpture, drawings, photography, decorative arts, and other artifacts.

Fast Exit
Carol Russell
Prescott, Arizona
Mixed Media Collage. 12" × 15". 2007.

My artwork is an exploration of the universal archetypal themes within the deeply personal, individual story. The collage and assemblage pieces tell stories in fragments, leaving the readers to fill in the undelineated with their own account, thus completing the narrative. This invitation to enter the story embraces the shared experience, or at least an experience, to which we are willing to be a witness.

Addiction touches everyone. I have family, friends, and acquaintances who have struggled with addiction. Through great effort, some have freed themselves from the clutch. Tragically, some have been lost. I hope that my art, as an expression of my own questioning and bereavement, will help to awaken some mutual recollection in the reader, thus contributing to the empathetic connection that links us all.

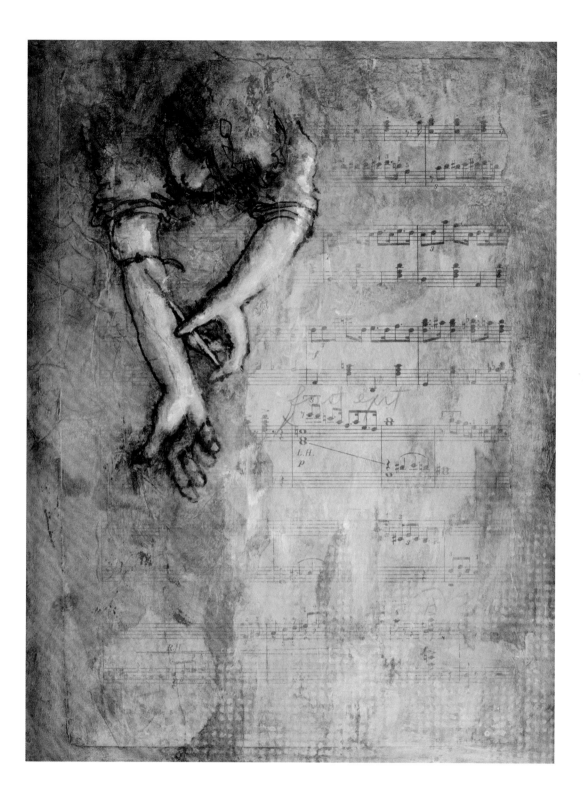

[17]

Relic
Anthony Santella
Teaneck, New Jersey
Mulberry Wood. 15" × 7" × 7". 2008.

My sculptural work draws on elements of both Catholic and African ritual art, particularly reliquaries and votive figures. In talking with someone very close to me about their past addiction, I was struck by their statement that all of their experiences from that time were tied up with drugs. To fully leave the bad parts of that life behind, they would have to forget good things also—friendships, excitement, moments of joy.

I imagined this reliquary, a container for something sacred and powerful, something to be treated carefully. It is a box to contain all of those things, good and bad. A place to keep them safe, not forgotten but put aside, preserved as a relic of one of the darker parts of the human experience, and a memento mori of a self that was but is no longer.

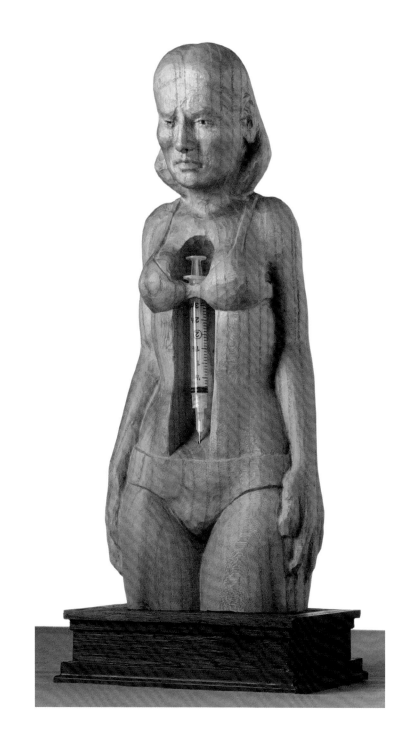

Valley of the Dolls, III
Patrick "STAR27" Deignan
St. Petersburg, Florida
Oil on Canvas. 20" × 20". 2003.

I have known the lost souls who haunt this world, searching for life in all the wrong places. I was one of them. So many wondrous people lose their purity to exploitation and hang a price tag on their bodies and souls. These are the subjects who populate my works.

The world is filled with bright lights to dazzle the eyes and fast ways to thrill the senses. My work reflects on the examples I have seen of the casualties of this twisted consumerism-based society we live in today. Those who stray into self-destruction seek basic needs—love, acceptance and happiness—and find them in dangerous places. I try to use my medium to undermine preconceptions and expose a society that praises wealth, possessions, and its own predetermined standards of beauty, at any cost.

The artist grew up in a loving home and began creating at a young age. Fearful of the world around him, he strayed into addiction. Always looking for the next thrill, he soon lost his health, peace of mind, and spirituality. Today he creates art about the darkness he has seen and the light he has found.

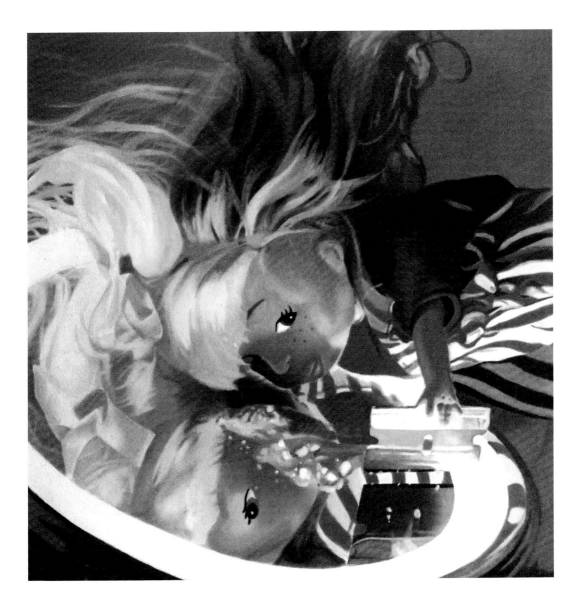

Number 11
Chris Ortiz
Baldwin City, Kansas
Photograph. 20" × 30". 2008.

For many drug users, addiction is the only escape from a bleak and hopeless world. Many addicts will go to any length to reach their "high"—separating themselves from the world because it holds no real value. For them, the only real value is the sensation they get from using drugs, even if it means inflicting pain on themselves to get high.

Number 11 depicts a young woman entrapped in the world of addiction, her eyes lacking the animation of life but showing instead the fine line between barely living and death.

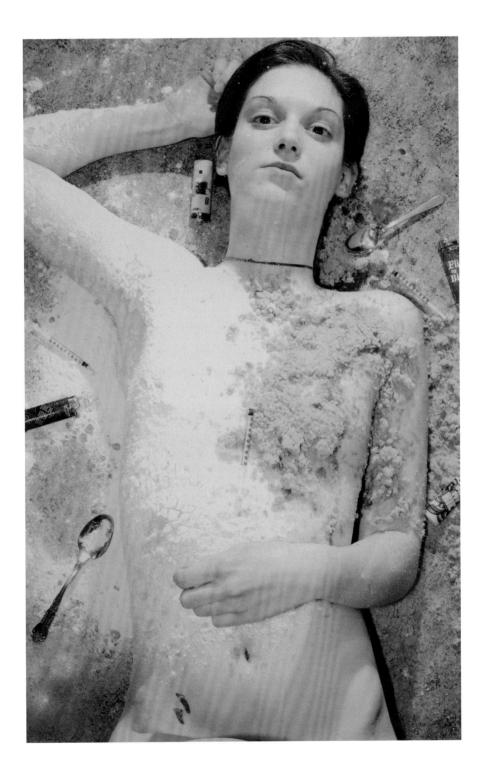

99 Bottles of Beer on the Wall
A Child's Introduction to Binge Drinking
(for Andy)
Michael C. Mendez
Martinsburg, West Virginia
Toned Silver Gelatin Print. 60" × 48". 2005.

99 Bottles of Beer on the Wall is from a larger body of work entitled "Occupation: Sinner," which has allowed me to explore my own admittedly self-destructive involvement with drugs and alcohol. The image focuses on factors that led me to abuse these substances. This particular piece calls attention to the way innocuous material in our formative years can shape our future attitudes. The work is dedicated to Andy Warhol (an allusion strengthened by the formal similarity to his *Three Coke Bottles*) and to a friend who died in a drunk driving accident.

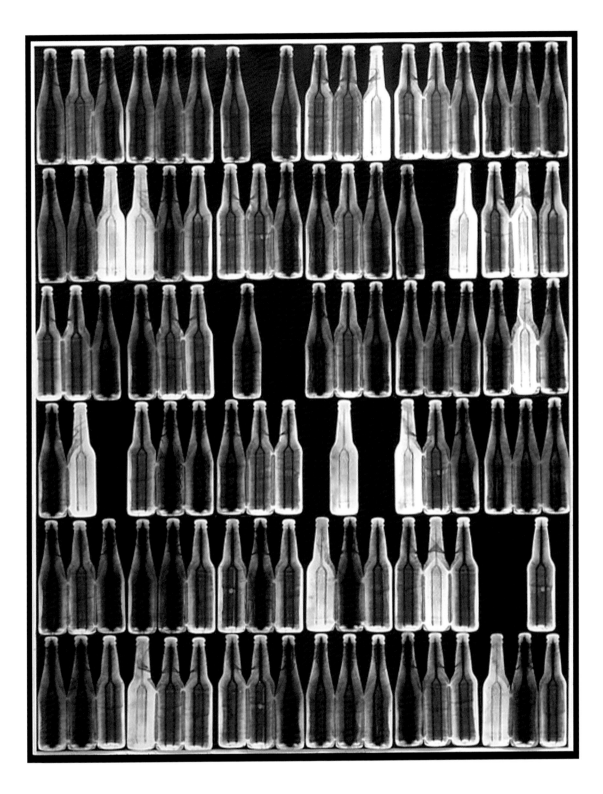

Nail Remover
Linda Lou Hubshman
Los Angeles, California
Acrylic and Ink on Wood. 23.5" × 11.5". 1998.

I have always been a jokester and was once a big drinker with many jokester drinking friends. My intention is to get a response through my paintings, whether it is just a quick passing chuckle or possibly a reminder to others of their own alcohol adventures. I think everyone has their own personal experience with addiction on a first- or second-hand basis.

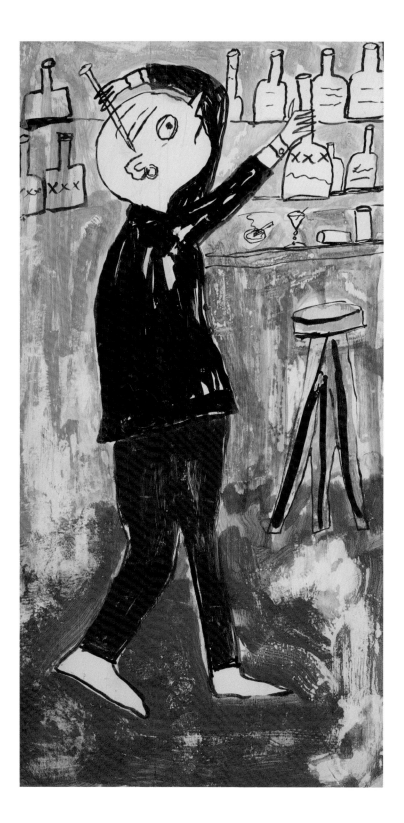

Urchin
Todd Lim
Stamford, Connecticut
Mixed Media. 12" × 12" × 12". 1993.

I have felt the prickling heat, the shivers and the shakes, what feels like a hundred needles jabbing through my skin at once, the chills that a winter coat on a hot summer's day cannot relieve. The signs begin with the tearing of watery eyes and a runny nose. I sneeze in rapid succession, gasping for air, gagging and choking when my throat closes up to a pinhole. The nausea, the retching, the vomiting with a bucket at arm's length—even that seems so far when all my strength has been drained. I urinate in a 2-liter plastic soda bottle rather than make the trip to the bathroom. I get the sweats that soak through my clothes, that press uncomfortably against my goose-pimpled skin. I jump or recoil from any human touch or the thought of taking a shower.

From the sleepless nights in bed, I toss and turn, kicking my legs. My feet rip the sheets on and off, running a marathon to reach the next worried and weary day. Then come the runs that burn the anus like an open faucet, spewing out like a sewer drain. These are the symptoms of heroin withdrawal in their various forms and stages, same old story through the ages. The only thing new is the body the addiction inhabits. What makes a person become a dirty and desperate wounded animal? Why am I like this?

Using the analogy and wordplay of the sea urchin and the street urchin, I realize that in a sea of possibilities, it is the choices I have made and the possibilities I can seize upon that will determine where and who I'll end up being.

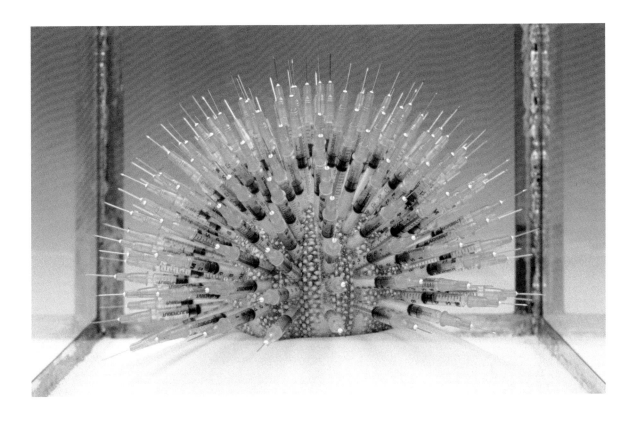

Blood Bubbles
Kristen Regan
Savannah, Georgia
Metallic Lambda C-Print. 20" × 24". 2007.

The association of intravenous drug use with la petite mort is inseparable. Using drugs, I had never felt more intense physical pleasure, but each time I also experienced a little death. The price I paid for such fleeting pleasure was a little death of my soul, morality, strength, and consequently the control of life in general.

I was fascinated with photographing fluids—intrinsically beautiful, delicate, and ephemeral. They spoke to me as if they were a visual narrative unfolding before my eyes. In altered states of mind, I lost my identity and tempted the ephemerality of life. *Blood Bubbles* was made ten years after I quit using drugs, which substantiates my transformation and represents my rebirth. Personal metamorphosis manifests within one's art. My photographs transformed from a physical documentation of my life into a theoretical questioning about life, death, creation, and rebirth.

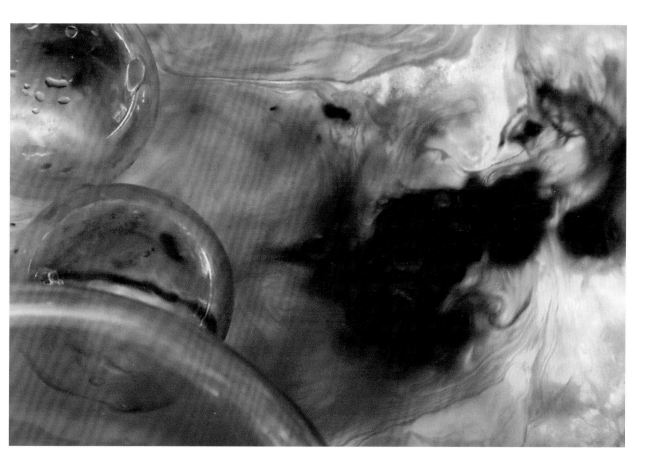

Boils
Abbey Aichinger
Avon, Indiana
Watercolor. 8" × 20". 2005.

As a kid, I dabbled pretty recklessly in drugs and alcohol but was smart enough (and lucky enough) to get out when I did. I have been fortunate never to have to deal with any serious addiction…the loneliness, the hopelessness, the denial. In this watercolor, *Boils*, I have tried to capture salient issues common to addiction.

I am a freelance illustrator with a Bachelor of Fine Arts degree from the Minneapolis College of Art and Design.

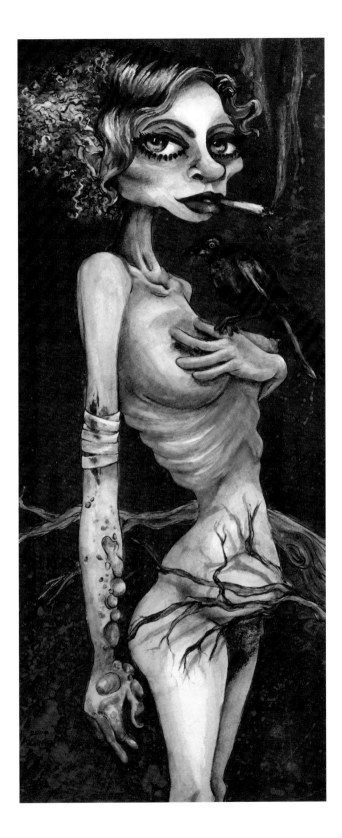

Prison
Brian Kelly
Fort Collins, Colorado
Digital Photograph. 11" × 17". 2007.

In every smoker's life there comes a day when they realize they cannot quit. It is a rare smoker who walks away the victor the first time they make a resolution to quit smoking. For most smokers, it is in this moment that they realize how they underestimated this substance and begin to comprehend the enormity of the "bad habit."

I feel it is important to communicate what it is like to be in the grip of an addiction. The fear and agony that drive an addiction are prisons that only bring pain and desperation. My intention is to help others understand what it is like to be an addict because I believe that the road to recovery would be more accessible if it were paved with understanding.

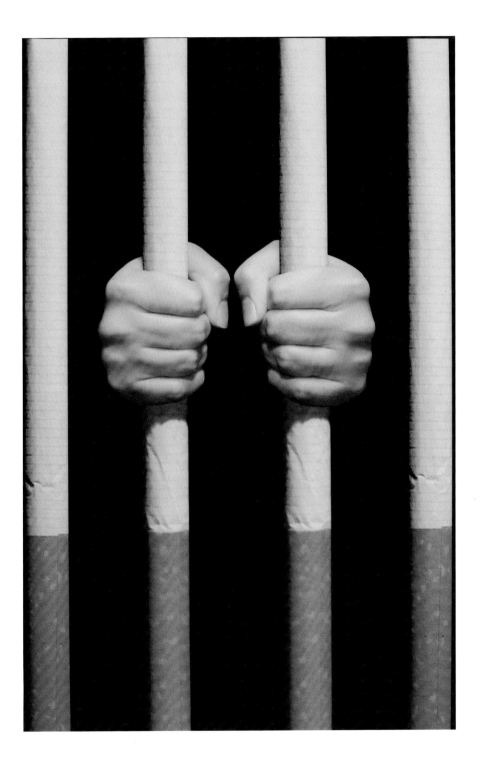

I'm Dying for a Smoke
Marie Balla
Arlington, Tennessee
Acrylic on Canvas. 12" × 12". 2008.

As a young adult, I grew up in a world where substance abuse was the norm. In high school I witnessed drunken peers throw back hard liquor between classes. In college I noticed pot smokers lounging in the same indented spot day after day. It's common knowledge to my age group to know which drugs have what effects on the body. TV, movies, magazines, video games, casual conversation—substance abuse is everywhere.

The one addiction society is numb to is tobacco smoking. "Death sticks," "cancer sticks," "tar fix" are all slang terms I've learned from cigarette smokers. Maybe it's the very slow, internal, unnoticeable effects of nicotine addiction that seem angelic in comparison to meth or coke addiction? I met an elderly man who smoked the majority of his life. He was diagnosed with emphysema and had to tote portable oxygen with him. Even that didn't stop him from smoking. He lit up despite his pain, embarrassment, and the knowledge he was making it all worse. That man resurfaced in my mind as I painted *I'm Dying for a Smoke.*

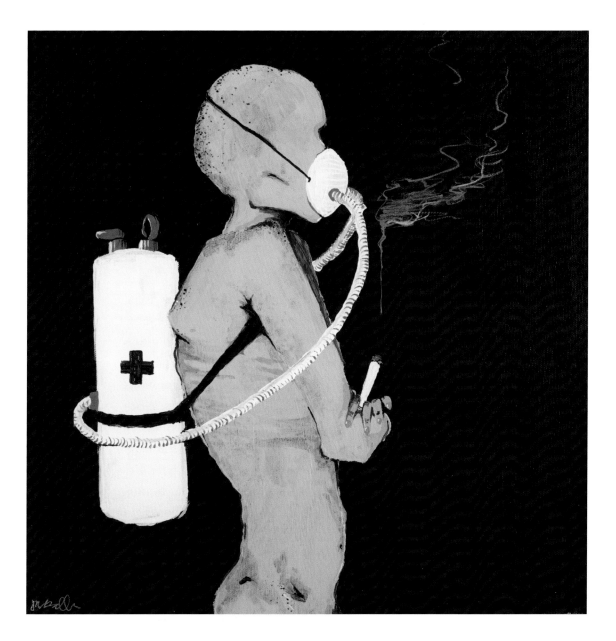

The Fabulosity of God
(and God created man in His own image)
Scott G. Brooks
Washington, D.C.
Oil on Canvas. 46" × 31". 2002.

The Fabulosity of God illustrates this biblical phrase: "God created man in His own image." Countering the belief that God's creations are without flaws, the painting presents the image of a man who is far from perfect yet is still whole and complete.

I often begin a painting without a clear vision of its meaning, and I end learning more about myself through the process. When I started painting *The Fabulosity of God*, I had a vague vision of a large man with missing limbs balanced on a barstool. The absence of limbs represents the loss of control.

As I spent time painting this man, his self-assured bearing began to emerge. Despite the undeniable damage his demons have waged, he persists in his strong resolve to maintain his behavior. He confidently exposes himself—the good, the bad, and the ugly—for the entire world to see, telling us we can either take him or leave him. The graphic imagery epitomizes the harmful choices and extreme sacrifices individuals make to feed their addictions.

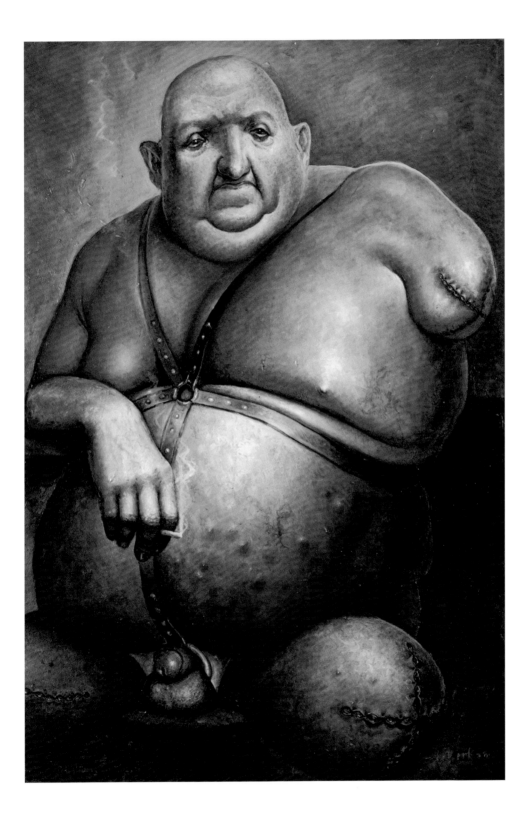

Recovery
Pedro de Valdivia
Seattle, Washington
Acrylic on Canvas. 24" × 30". 2008.

My work is intended to connect visually without words. The power of pictures speaks even to those who do not know how to read. One of my objectives is to characterize the psychological entrapments of drug addiction.

My art is a patchwork of detailed symbolism for understanding the cruel bondage of drugs. The vibrant heart symbolizes the center of our personality, intuition, and the core of our being. I have felt chained and held down in my life, but against all odds I found my voice through art. Expressing myself through art provides the way to deal with personal difficulties. The power to imagine is a way to grow through harsh realities.

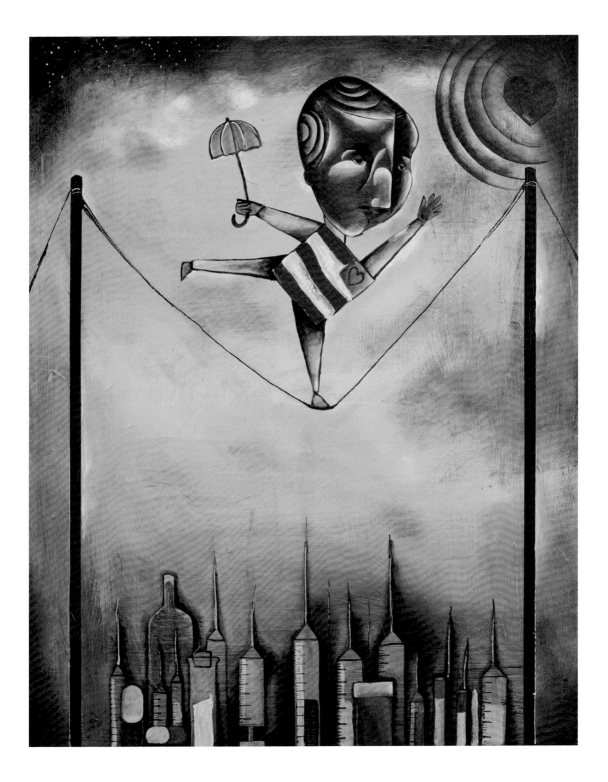

Reincarnation into a Hallucinogenic World
Aradhna Tandon
Haryana, India
Oil on Canvas. 34.5" × 48.5". 2005.

Two lives—desolate, confused, and morose—have submerged their worlds into the false hope of alcohol. While they wish to see themselves reincarnated (as suggested by the ritualistic "thread" around the man's ear) into original innocence, the truth of their lives is mirrored in the bottles. The static-ness of the visual imagery suggests the unmoving stillness of the lives depicted.

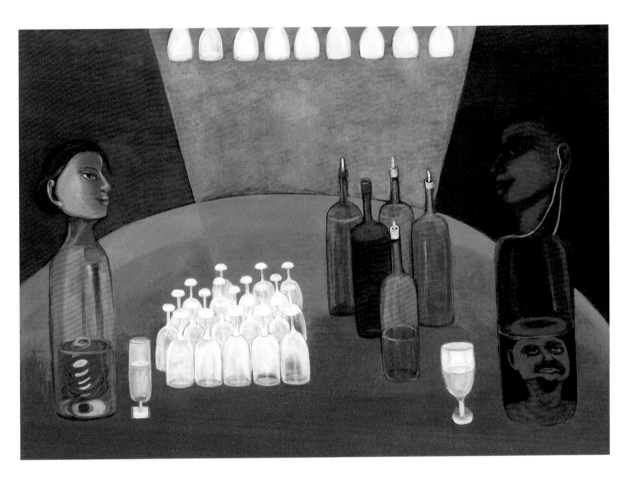

Trigger
Brian Kelly
Fort Collins, Colorado
Digital Photograph. 11" × 17". 2007.

I am a recovering addict, and addiction has served a very important role in my life. Addictions are coping mechanisms. They are often formed early in life to protect the addict from something. Addiction eventually becomes a destroyer that consumes everything in its path. This work addresses my struggle with and feelings about alcoholism, from which I am recovering.

Being able to identify your "triggers" is beneficial to an alcoholic. Although the term refers to a situation, emotion, or state of mind that initiates the compulsion to take the first drink, it has been all too evident in my recovery that the first drink will ultimately lead to death and is essentially suicide. For an alcoholic, to drink is to die. I wish this was merely a clever metaphor, but it is not.

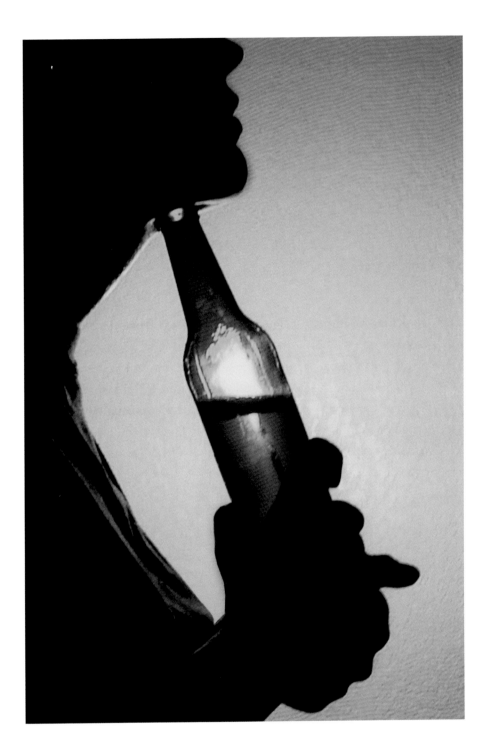

Now That You're Gone,
I Can't Apologize
Robb Siverson
Fargo, North Dakota
Gelatin Silver Print. 16" × 20". 2003.

Now That You're Gone, I Can't Apologize is from an ongoing series that started in 2002. With this particular body of work, subjects are allowed to wander in obscure, sometimes uncomfortable situations. With drawn-out titles, evoking an intimate frame of mind, a variety of aspects concerning the human psyche is captured...A unique chemical process is then applied to the photograph, giving a painterly quality to the image, making it a truly unique, "one of a kind" piece.

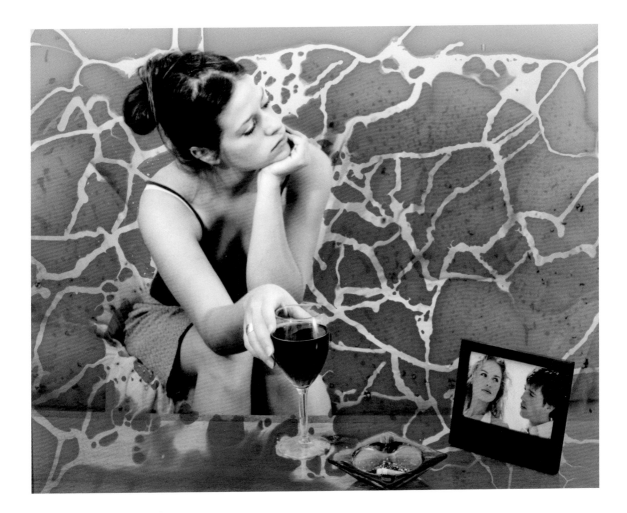

[47]

Toy Soldier
Deborah Feller
New York, New York
Charcoal and White Chalk Pencils on Sepia Paper.
30" × 20". 2006.

As an addictions professional for the past 33 years, I have heard many stories of childhood neglect and abuse from alcoholics and other addicts in facilities where I have worked and in my private practice. Twelve years ago, when I began seriously studying art, I realized I could use my artistic abilities to share what I had learned about the toll that drugs and alcohol, and childhood neglect and abuse (especially incest) take on children. By drawing (and painting) my clients' stories, I could increase awareness about these problems, while at the same time honoring my clients' struggles.

Toy Soldier shows a 7-year-old boy entranced by his play while his alcoholic mother lies passed out drunk on the floor. The boy grew up to become an alcoholic but now in recovery is a successful businessman, a life that renders invisible the neglect he suffered as a child.

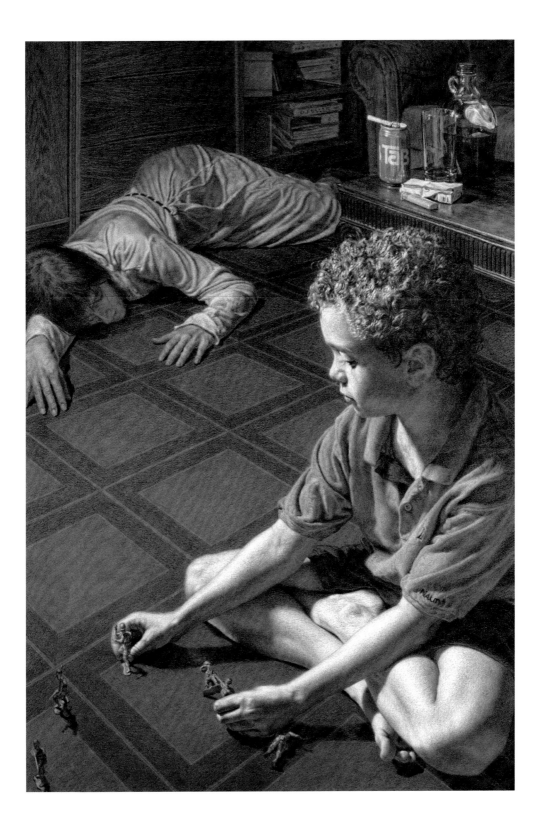

ō'vər-thə-koun'tər
Robyn L. Gray
Denver, Colorado
Ceramic, Slip Cast, Acrylic Paint, Paste Wax.
24" × 17" × 6". 2007.

Sculpture, more specifically clay, is the way I interpret and understand my surroundings. Since childhood I have realized that addiction was a part of everyday life—from family dinner to the overwhelming emotions tied to abuse and suicide. These everyday circumstances became so intertwined in my culture and relationships that I began to see them as normal.

Now as an artist, I find these memories and emotions to be as powerful today as they were years ago. Through the assembly and manipulation of my art, I attempt to inject feelings of fear, powerlessness, and anger while also layering them with feelings of hope, humor, and redemption. Addiction can happen to anyone, and that struggle inspires me to create art that hopefully leads to healing and helps to create a dialogue of understanding.

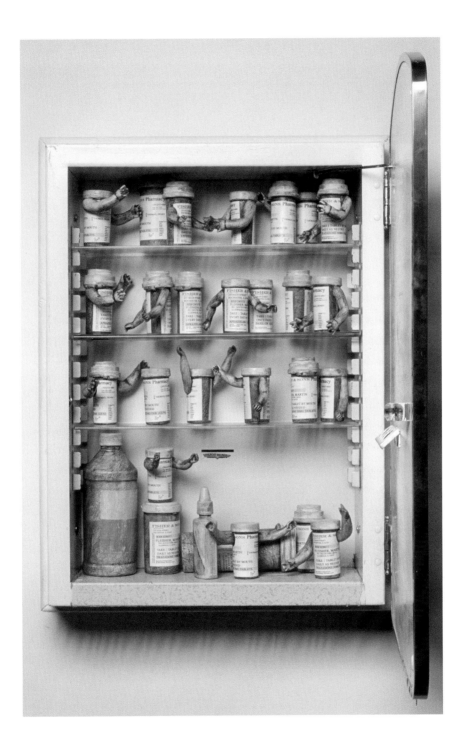

Three Square
Stephen Cummings
Tempe, Arizona
Pastel on Hardboard Panel. 10" × 10". 2008.

Three Square addresses the incredibly casual approach to drug use that abounds in our culture. The solution to every ailment, however minor, seems to come in the form of a pill. Consumers are constantly bombarded by a slew of medications with the promise of relief from conditions both age-old and newly named. Doctors peddle drugs with hardly a glance at a patient's symptoms, so prescription drugs could scarcely be easier to come by, and ever fewer of us think twice before popping whichever pill will alleviate whatever problem happens to occur. Furthermore, recreational use, increasingly popular, is a symptom and example of the overt flippancy that harbors the dangerous potential for addiction.

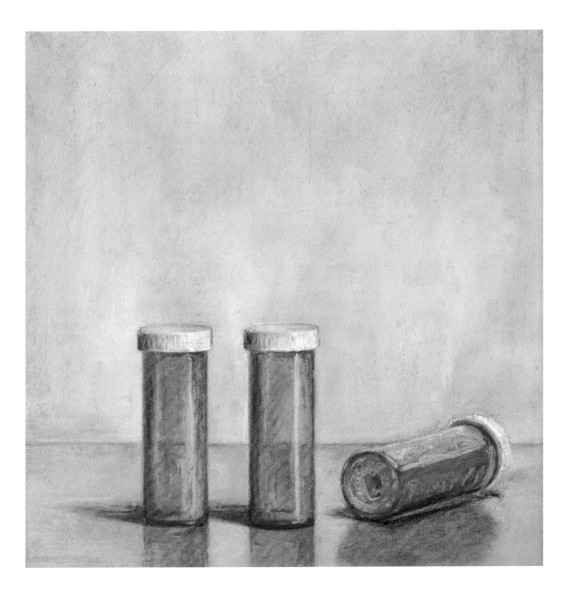

Two Triple Cheese
Marnie Spencer
Bolinas, California

Acrylic, Ink, and Pencil on Canvas. 16" × 7". 2007.

Nepenthe is a drinck of soverayne grace,

Devized by the Gods, for to asswage

Harts grief, and bitter gall away to chace

Edmund Spenser, *The Faerie Queene*

Two Triple Cheese projects the mundane glitter of everyday addiction. Glamor is not needed; base needs and instincts plus pop culture iconism are enough. Heroin, coke, dope, booze, nicotine, Big Macs, moronic ideologies, a fool's draw to an inside straight—this stuff helps us to feel good or to forget what doesn't.

Can art provide a cure? As Jung stated, art is itself addictive ("Every form of addiction is bad, no matter whether the narcotic be alcohol, morphine, or idealism."), and artists can't help that. If you're not part of the solution, you're an artist. As William Congreve noted, however, "Music hath charms to soothe the savage breast." So maybe art can foster enough positive or palliative feelings to break addictive chains. Winston Churchill (*Painting as Pastime*) thought that painting restored his psychic equilibrium, provided solace, and was "a companion, . . . a friend that makes no undue demands, excites no exhausting pursuits, keeps faithful pace even with feeble steps, and holds her canvas as a screen between us and the envious eyes of Time."

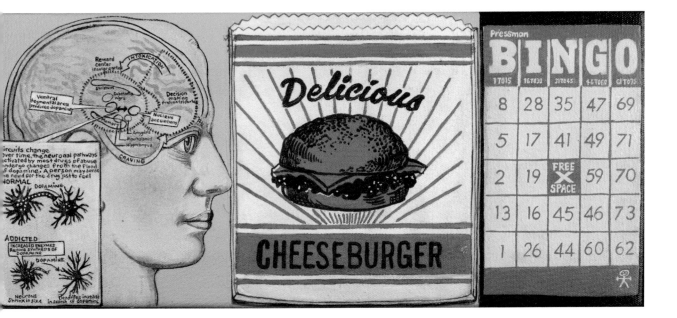

Obesity
Joseph Barbaccia
Potomac Falls, Virginia
Mixed Media, Polychromed Clay, Stainless Steel.
3.5" × 10" × 4.5". 2006.

Eating is one of life's needs that can go awry. *Obesity* attempts to communicate the imbalance and destructiveness of a typical eating disorder. The juxtaposition of oozy, flabby flesh being forced through the cold, sharp edges of a stainless steel cheese grater creates an image that unsettles the mind and offers a different perspective.

Herein lies the value of art, a portal that allows us to see past our own worldly constructs into the unknown. Art lets us create socially acceptable objects (artwork), exposing hitherto unexplored pathways of understanding. Art is the window both into and out of oneself, revealing new viewpoints and discoveries.

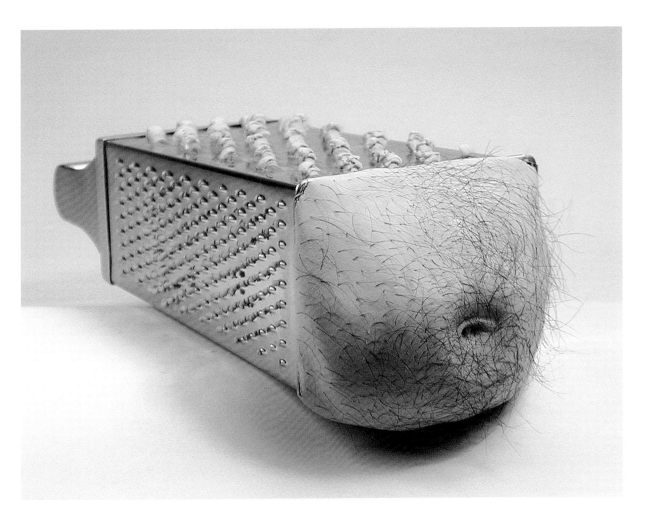

Addiction
Camille Rogers
Modesto, California
Digital Print. 8" × 8". 2008.

Addiction represents my own personal struggle with food. I had poor nutrition, ate unhealthy food, and my health suffered because of it. In this image, the roots represent the darkness we create within ourselves—how addiction takes hold of us. Addiction prevents us from moving on and succeeding in life. We must cut ourselves free from addiction by using love and the strength of our will.

There was not one specific incident that caused me to want to get better...mostly I was tired of being a prisoner of my addiction. I am getting better. Although some days are more challenging than others, the answer is to just keep going and never give up on yourself. I am the one person who can stop my addictive behaviors.

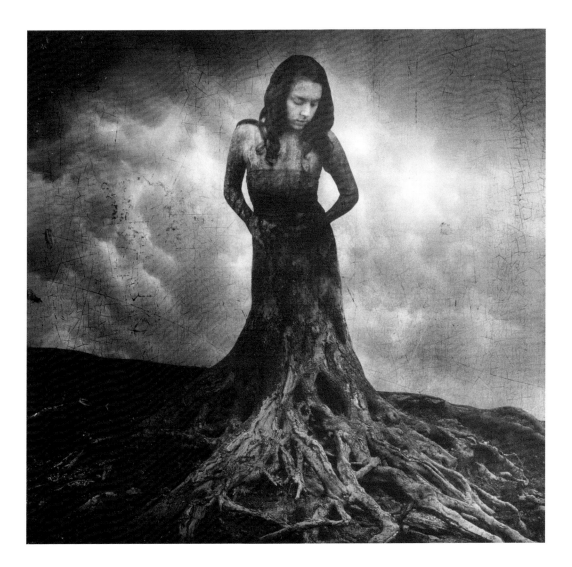

Matthew
Matthew Beals
Frederick, Maryland
(Submitted by Callyn Beals)
Photograph. 5" × 7". 2007.

This is a photograph of my brother, Matthew Beals, who died at the age of 25 from an addiction to methamphetamine and from AIDS on June 14, 2007. He was loving and caring—everything one could ask for in a brother—until he became addicted to meth.

This self-portrait, taken by him in San Francisco, represents the speed with which he lived his life and the drug that eventually ended it.

by Callyn Beals

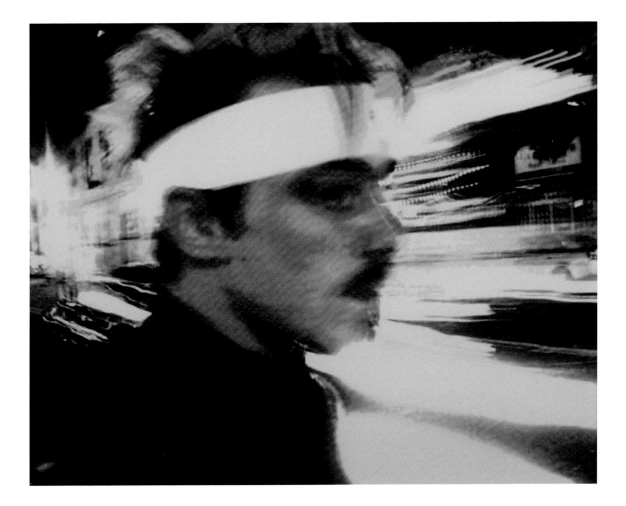

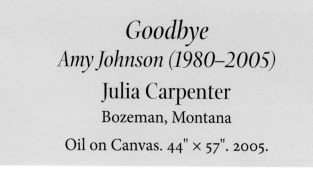

Goodbye
Amy Johnson (1980–2005)
Julia Carpenter
Bozeman, Montana
Oil on Canvas. 44" × 57". 2005.

My sister, Amy, was a bright, engaging, and beautiful young woman. Her promising life turned tragic when she became addicted to heroin in her teens. For years Amy struggled to gain control over her addiction. While I was in the military serving overseas, my family reported that Amy was attending college and by all appearances was doing quite well.

Amy died of a heroin overdose at the age of 24. After her death, I read her journal entries, went through her belongings, and made discoveries about her life I could never have imagined. As I learned more about the darkness of her life and the masks of conventionality she wore, my grief intensified and my reality was shaken. After losing my sister to heroin addiction, I questioned everything I once knew about her. My painting of Amy is based on a photograph taken of her two months before her death.

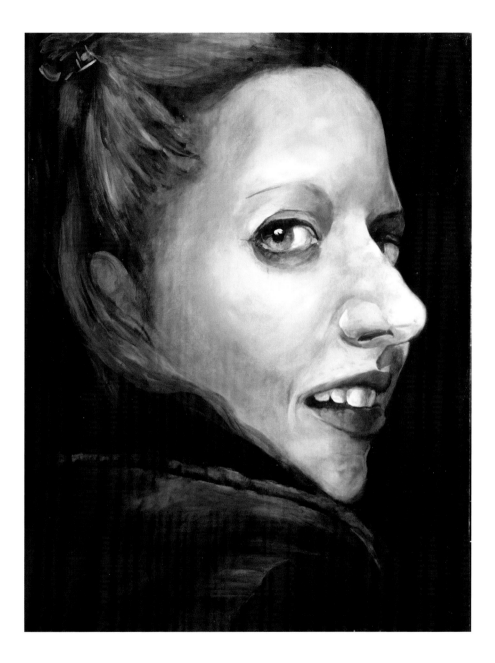

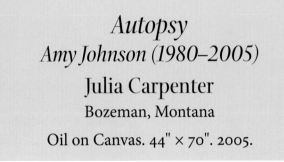

Autopsy
Amy Johnson (1980–2005)
Julia Carpenter
Bozeman, Montana
Oil on Canvas. 44" × 70". 2005.

This book contains two portraits of my late sister, Amy Johnson, who died from heroin addiction. The paintings are excerpts from a larger series of ten portraits that document the persistence of my grief over her premature death. The creation of this body of work allowed me to explore her loss as I tried to reconcile my memories about her with the harsh realities of her life lost to addiction. The portraits reflect my ensuing anger over her death, my confusion about her life, and my questions about the physical death of the human body. Using the template of the human face, I discovered within the genre of portraiture the ability to go beyond the traditional to express the unspeakable.

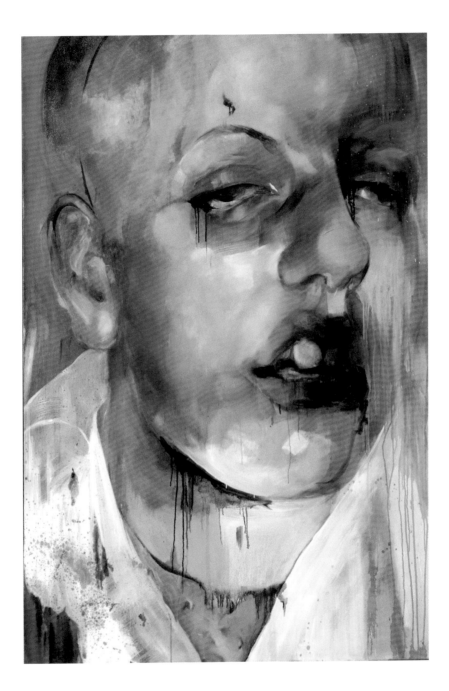

The Chains of Addiction
Jose F. Garcia
Miami, Florida

Photograph. 8.5" × 11". 2008.

As a practicing mental health professional, I deal with the theme of drug addiction and recovery on a regular basis. As an artist, my objective in *The Chains of Addiction* is to illustrate the feelings of despair, loneliness, and apathy that are hallmarks of chemical addiction. My work depicts the pain and isolation of drug addiction without romanticizing it.

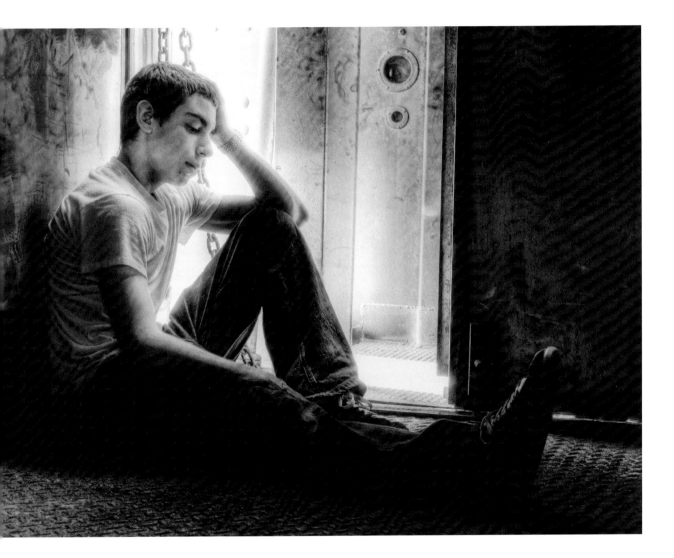

Lifeline
Claudia Flynn
Wakefield, Rhode Island
C-Print and Red Thread Stitching. 32" × 15". 2004.

After I recovered from a particularly bad bout with a depressive episode, the importance of maintaining personal life support systems became imperative to me—a way to manage my own life with struggles in tow. That is key to maintaining my own recovery and optimal wellness.

With this in mind, I made the two-dimensional piece *Lifeline*. I placed my hand and arm on an office copy machine. From that single copy, the black and white image was transferred to Photoshop software and digitally elongated for emphasis. The final and essential element was the stitching up of the "lifeline" (as referenced in palmistry). This red-threaded stitch resembles a surgical suture employed to treat and heal a wound. The hand gesture is cautiously optimistic, signifying hope that the pain is lessening.

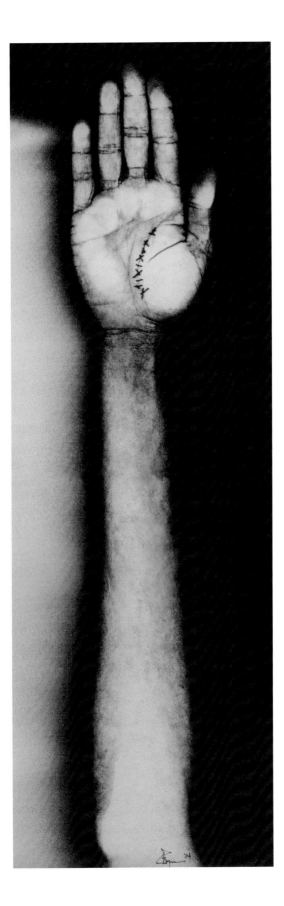

[69]

Flower Child
Charlotte Huntley
Lafayette, California
Watercolor. 22" × 30". 2001.

This painting is named for the "flower children" of the 1960s in San Francisco. This emaciated young man lives in a village in Thailand. Judging from the skeletal condition of his body, I presume he lives on opium. He made this trashy hat and decorated it with flowers. He evidently made the opium pipe too. There is a lot of talent going "down the tube" or "up in smoke." I have no idea what the blue thing is hanging from his hat. I tell people it is probably a cell phone to call for more opium.

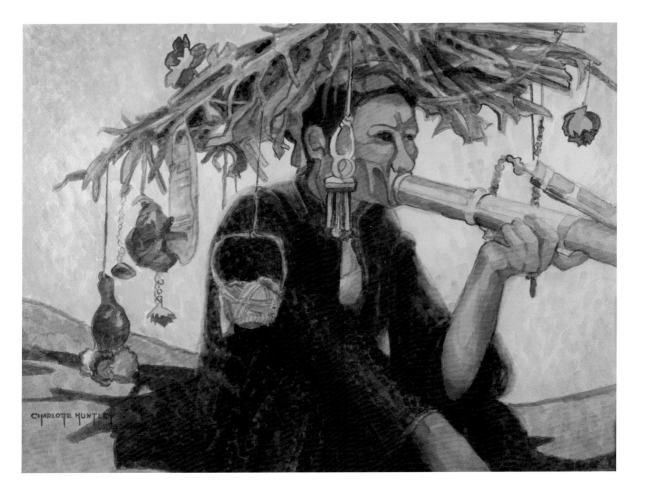

What Is a Poison? What Is a Remedy? Marijuana

Nash Hyon

Wilton, Connecticut

Oil on Canvas. 72" × 48". 1998.

My husband smoked in his twenties but then quit. He died of lung cancer at the age of 61; the cancer metastasized to his brain and bones. Why was it a problem for his doctors to give him morphine for his pain? Did they think he would become addicted? For me, this was another form of drug abuse—withholding palliative care from patients who truly need it.

My painting is intended to generate discussion concerning the dangers and, in some cases, controlled benefits of substances in the hope that people will think and ask questions about these important issues.

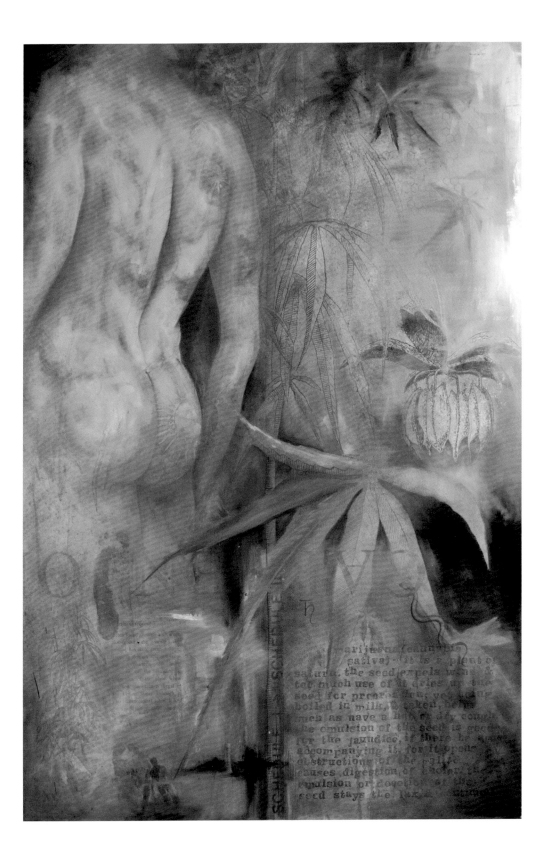

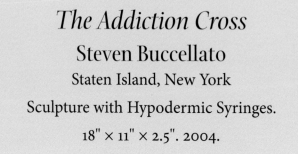

The Addiction Cross
Steven Buccellato
Staten Island, New York

Sculpture with Hypodermic Syringes.

18" × 11" × 2.5". 2004.

The Addiction Cross is an experimental artwork that uses unconventional media (hypodermic syringes) to explore a growing problem in our society: the use of intravenous drugs. Drug use creates and increases one's exposure to HIV/AIDS through the use of dirty needles. This situation has caused some communities to develop needle exchange programs to help fight the war on drugs and limit the spread of the epidemic. What it doesn't do is help cure the addict.

Much like the spiritual devotee, the addict takes the communion of their new god each time they exchange the old syringe with the new and use a drug to get "high." A "medium with a message," the addiction cross is both delivery method and a representation of this new god. Society's fear of disease and the struggle to come to terms with HIV/AIDS, drug use, and addiction cannot be stifled by politicians or the church. The line between addiction and belief has blurred. One can feel the pain and hardship of the faithful (the addict), as seen in the anguish of the corpus upon the cross. One must find one's way to fight addiction either through spirituality or through active involvement.

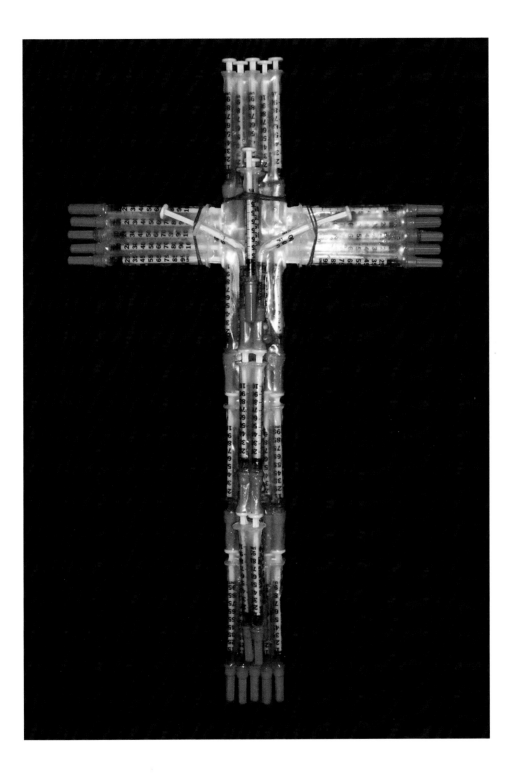

The Addiction Savior
Erich W. March
Baltimore, Maryland
Acrylic on Canvas. 20" × 24". 2007.

As a funeral director in Baltimore City, where more than 10 percent of the population is drug dependent, I witness firsthand the deadly effects and devastation of addiction. Whether the addictive substances are drugs, alcohol, or cigarettes, the long-term abuse of these body-destroying chemicals has only one outcome—premature death. While many seek help and enter treatment, the reality is that the relapse rate for drug addiction is extremely high, indicating that the addictive drug hunger is more than many wanting permanent relief can overcome.

As an artist, I painted *The Addiction Savior* to depict the redemptive healing power of God as administered by a non-condemning, burden-bearing collaborator who loves the addicted beyond their faults and joins with them in the struggle to overcome their addiction. Encouraging confidence in God's unconditional love and in an addict's faith coupled with determination has sometimes proven to be an effective recovery treatment when all else fails.

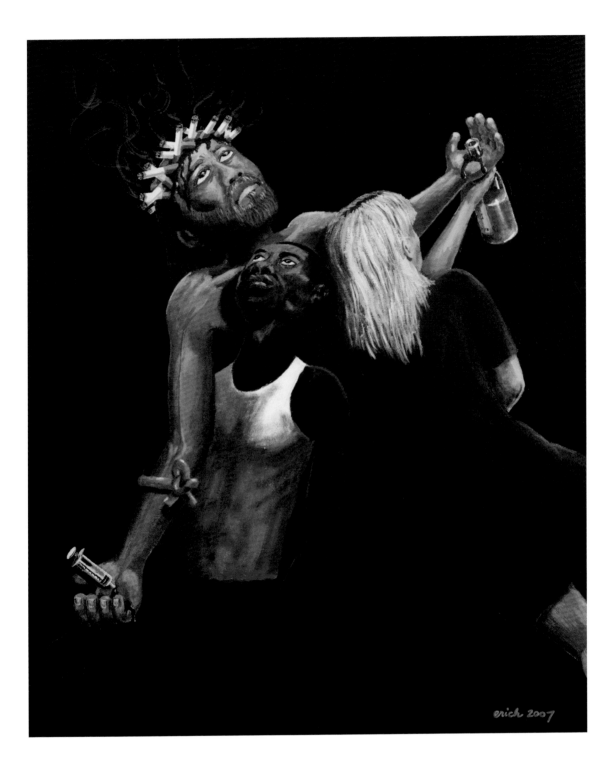

erich 2007

My Kingdom for a Horse
Marianela de la Hoz
San Diego, California

Egg Tempera, Goldleaf on Board. 4" × 4". 2006.

As an artist, I have devoted myself to depicting the dark side of the human being, the Mr. Hyde who coexists with Dr. Jekyll. This dark side is present, and although we cannot see it easily, this is where we can find a very deep and obscure well into which those who abuse drugs and alcohol have fallen. They can liberate themselves only through a rehabilitation program and with an iron will.

My Kingdom for a Horse represents the desperation felt by the fallen. They have lost their way in this horrific hell of drugs, thinking in a self-deceptive way that using drugs would make them feel better. Using drugs allows them to run away from problems or unpleasant realities; allows them to pretend they are "royalty," perhaps becoming a king or a wealthy child living in better times. The character depicted in my painting longs for release from the darkness that lives within him. He has lost battles, friends, family, work, perhaps everything. He is at the point of sacrificing his own life just to return to the light once again.

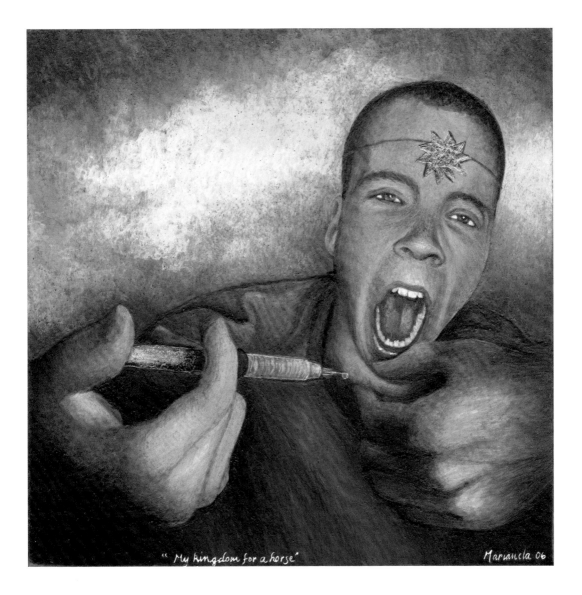

"My kingdom for a horse"

Mariancla 06

In the Eyes of ...
Joseph Heidecker
Bellport, New York
Found Photograph, Beads. 21" × 26". 2004.

I grew up in an alcoholic family. I became attracted to certain outrageous and less conventional types of people who were also alcoholics. As alcohol starts to take a seat of importance throughout the week, the soul's energy starts to drain away. The mood is always up and down. Concerns for other individuals, ideas, and duties slowly lose their importance. The daily routine continues, seemingly normal on the surface, but the attitude that develops gets bleaker and less joyful. Internal thoughts become skewed, and interpretation of one's surroundings and relationships to others becomes more strained and distorted. One's personal image becomes transformed. Self-respect is low and regard for one's behavior is not important.

In the Eyes of ... can be interpreted as a metaphor for how toxic reality becomes from the alcoholic's perspective.

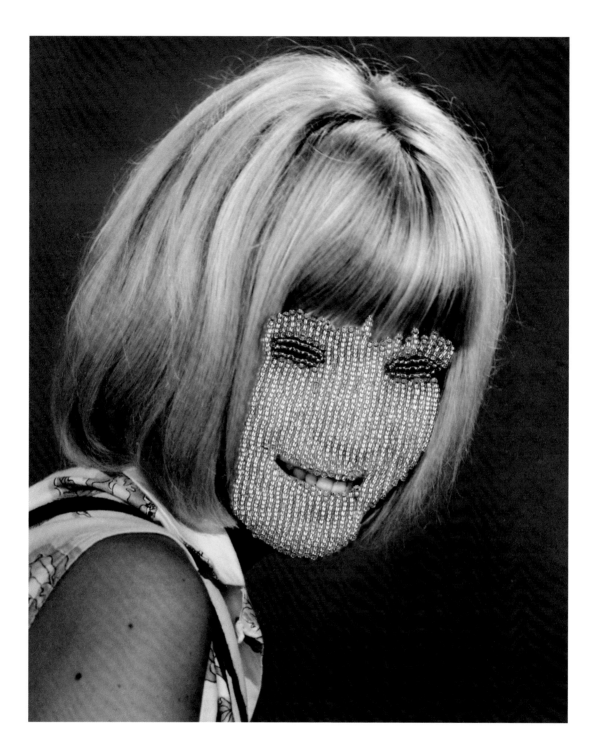

Living Hell
Jacquelyn Bond
Portland, Oregon
Watercolor. 12" × 16". 2008.

I have illustrated the drug abuse that seems to go unnoticed. In my life, I have been affected by illegal and legal drugs. Growing up with a mother who was addicted to alcohol and prescription drugs, I know all too well how it is swept under the rug; when the addict is confronted, the excuse is always "the doctor gave me these, so I need them." My mother is now 53 years old and is in jail for her fourth "driving while intoxicated" offense.

Children increasingly abuse prescription drugs and do not see it as a problem since prescription drugs are legal. Our entire country is under the prescription medicine cloud—our most pressing drug epidemic. I hope that the future brings this to light and that it will be treated as aggressively as addiction to illegal drugs.

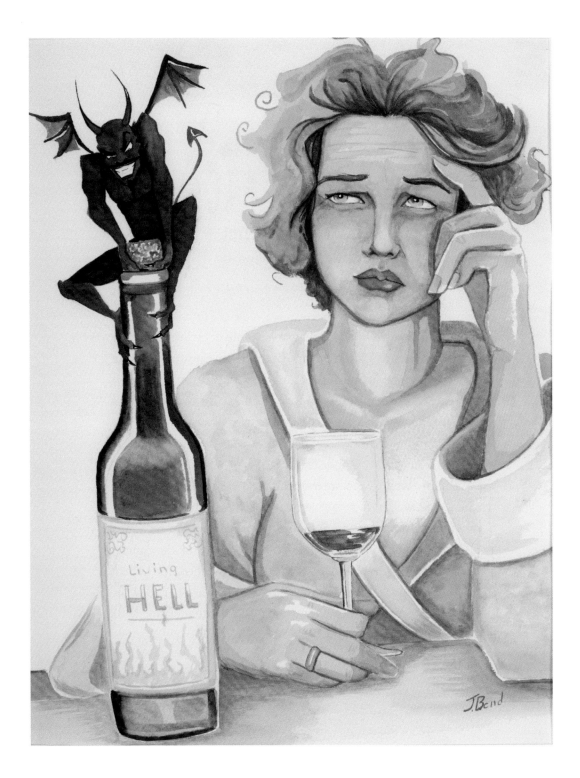

River of Tears
Carmen Beecher
Satellite Beach, Florida
Oil and Collage. 11" × 14". 2008.

My father gave up his fight against alcoholism by taking his own life. How many rivers of tears have been shed because of addiction? Each tear in the background of my painting represents a family member whose demise was hastened by his or her own addictions, but the focus of the painting is my father. The crow represents Death, and the bottle is spilling blood because his death was a violent one.

In the *River of Tears* are those most affected by his act: his children, wife, and mother. We were left with pain, shock, and sorrow, but as we matured and the trauma of his suicide became a more distant memory, anger and disappointment became the compelling emotions. The thirsty river is not yet quenched, for we have lived to see the family disease rear its ugly head again, and we are justifiably terrified for our loved ones fighting the terrible battle against the demons of addiction.

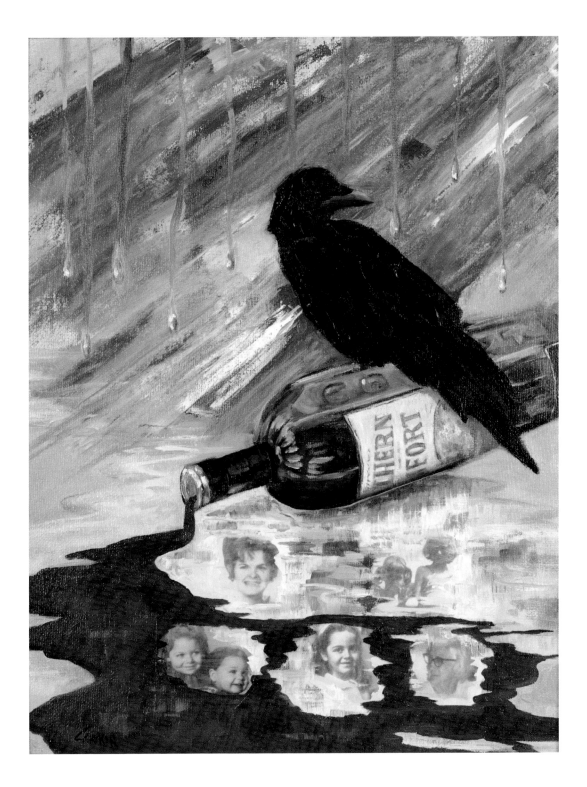

Empowered
Jill Nonnemacher
Mansfield, Texas
Acrylic on Canvas. 24" × 36". 2008.

As I am an artist, trained psychotherapist, and certified alcohol and substance abuse counselor, following my passion has given me the opportunity to paint, exhibit my art, and help others to express themselves through art and therapy.

Empowered represents the struggles and adverse consequences one may have experienced with alcohol. My goal is to visually make a strong impression on the viewer by stirring emotions. Connecting to my art, those who have abused or become dependent on alcohol may perhaps see themselves in *Empowered*, which hopefully will stimulate a responsive action to help them put an end to their destructive behaviors and stop the cycle of addiction.

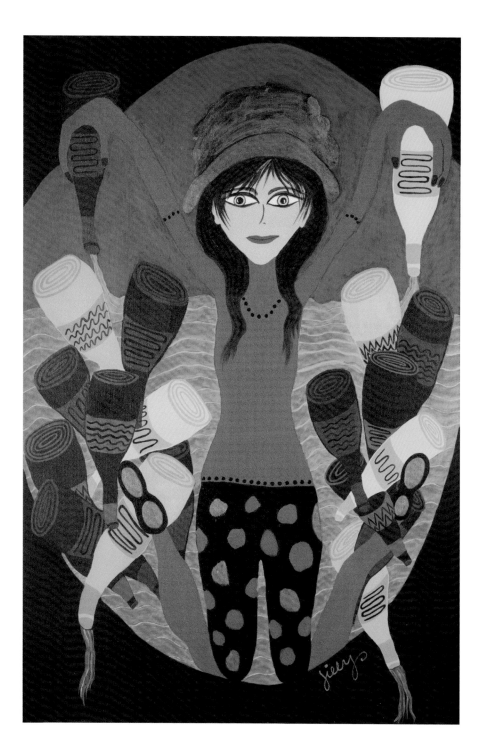

The Ticket to Recovery
Todd Lim
Stamford, Connecticut
Silkscreen on Board. 24" × 36". 2002/2007.

As a patient at a methadone clinic, I have tried to free myself from heroin dependency. I believed I could eventually wean myself from methadone, too. Gradually, I dropped my dose down to 8 mg but could not withstand the pain of withdrawal. Because my constitution is not strong enough at this time, I find myself back where I started. The doctor at the clinic told me to think of myself as a diabetic who would need insulin. This might be more comforting, if not for the stigma and handicaps attached to such a circumstance. As a methadone user, I cannot help but feel that society judges and scrutinizes the recovering addict as a pariah, a potential risk and liability. This is understandable, although it makes it much more difficult to be accepted in re-entering society as a functioning and responsible person.

In my struggles to find my identity and a place in this world, I have created this artwork. It is based on my daily experiences with the clinic as well as my meetings in groups and with my counselor. They have been an inspiration, guiding force, and safe harbor in helping me to rebuild and accept a part of myself.

By creating this artwork, I am trying to appeal to society about the need for awareness and compassion. The more we understand the causes that perpetuate substance abuse, the better we will be able to deal and cope with the problems, the solutions, and their effects.

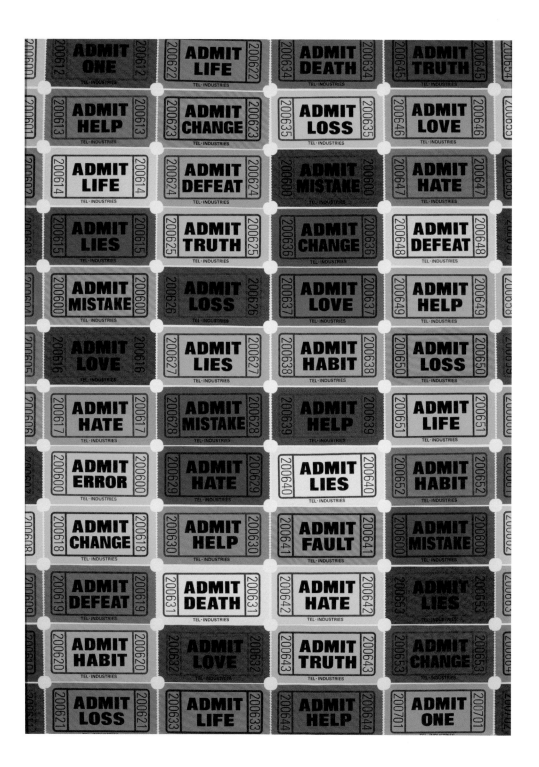

Too Many Cigarettes
Fausta Facciponte
Mississauga, Ontario, Canada
Pencil Drawing. 8.5" × 12". 2008.

Children who live in homes where they are exposed to cigarette smoking are at higher risk of following that path. *Too Many Cigarettes* portrays a cartoonish child smoking two cigarettes at once. The child also appears ready for a party, symbolizing the fun of childhood but simultaneously hinting at the predisposition for drug addiction.

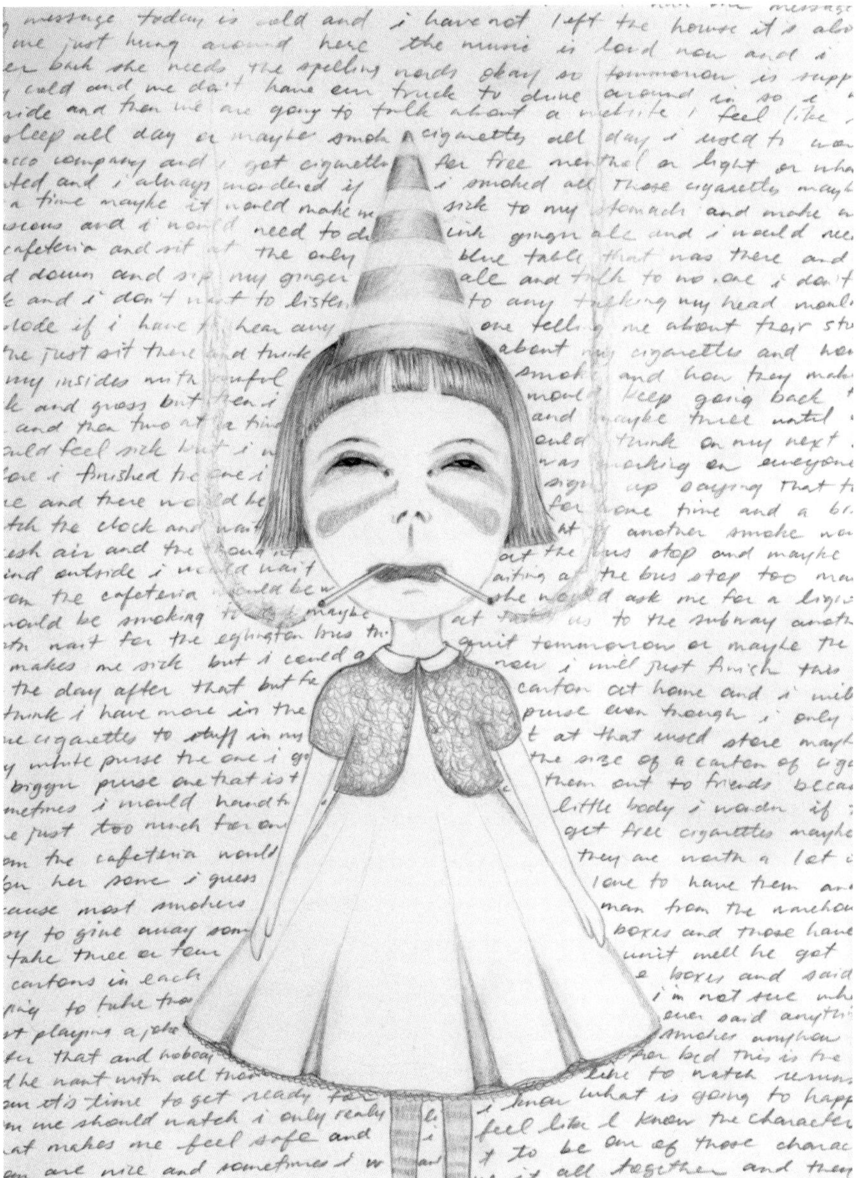

The Smokinhalator
Kim Carr Valdez
Brooklyn, New York

Sculpture (found and altered commercially available parts). 96" × 28" × 42". 2004.

The inspiration for this false invention was New York State's Indoor Clean Air Act of 2003. I am a former smoker myself, with loved ones who still smoke, so this legislation led to many passionate debates. Some individuals did lose personal freedom, while others gained the freedom not to inhale toxic second-hand smoke. Because of increasing public awareness within the course of a few decades, smoking cigarettes changed from an activity one could do socially anywhere to an addiction—a forbidden activity with a very negative and isolating social stigma.

The Smokinhalator is a prototype of a concept for a self-contained air filtration system that would enable the smoker to smoke cigarettes indoors despite recent legislation in many states and communities prohibiting this activity. The mission is to enable the smoker to smoke in a variety of public and private locations, including bars, office buildings, and at home. A personal kit, including a mask and cigarette holder, would be available for purchase by the customer at area retailers.

The Smokinhalator is a sculptural installation, which has now been disassembled because of difficulty in finding both a legal and an appropriate venue for its display and use.

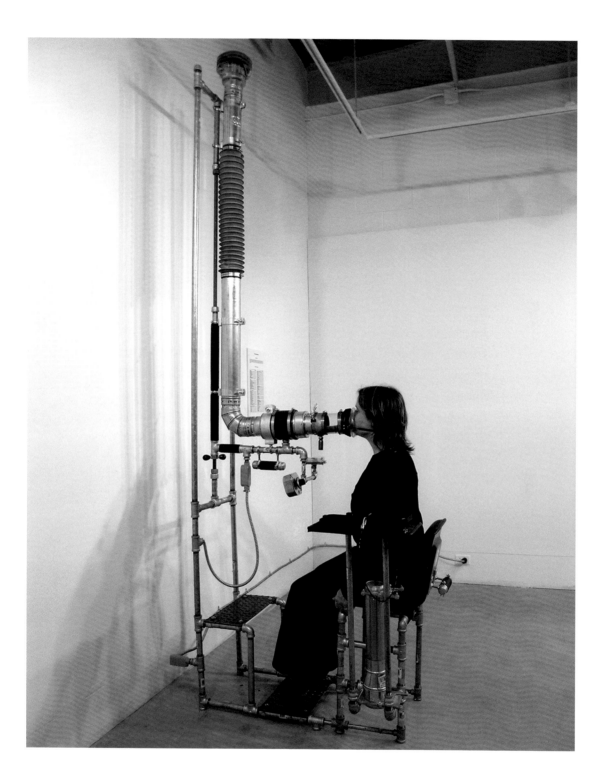

Trapped among Whom?
Marilyn Rodriguez-Behrle
Philadelphia, Pennsylvania
Pen, Oil Pastel on Cardboard. 11" × 14". 2007.

I work at a psychiatric hospital, which has greatly influenced my artwork. Addiction and other issues related to mental health are primary images reflected in my art, which I refer to as "haunting images." *Trapped among Whom?* is part of my series of masked figures—homeless people with untreated psychiatric problems. These lost souls live in many communities throughout our country.

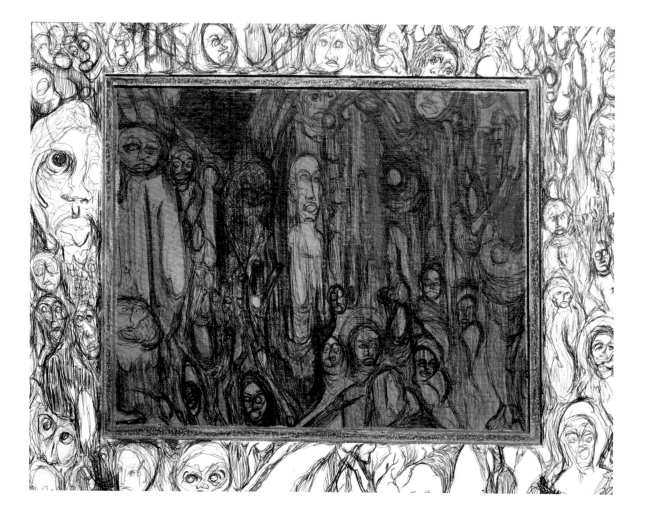

Prodigal Son
Karen Swenholt
Falls Church, Virginia
Aqua Resin. 86" × 54" × 38". 2007.

Prodigal's Dream

If a father could be perfect
If a father could love long.
If a father could forgive
Though I had taken a bath in wrong,
If my father could weep sometimes because I had gone away,
Taken three steps, then dove down into every kind of play,
If he would only long for me in an almost woman kind of way,
Then maybe I'd come back to him someday.

If a father's love could be strong enough to bathe in and come out
   clean,
Father's love bond enough to call me home again,
If he would cover me with feathers and incubate my good,
Shine, burnish it until it shined nearly as he could,
He'd lift my head with steady hands,
Tell me my life's worth living, that he loves me as I am.
Then I'd stretch across that empty canyon's span.

I'd come back to him.

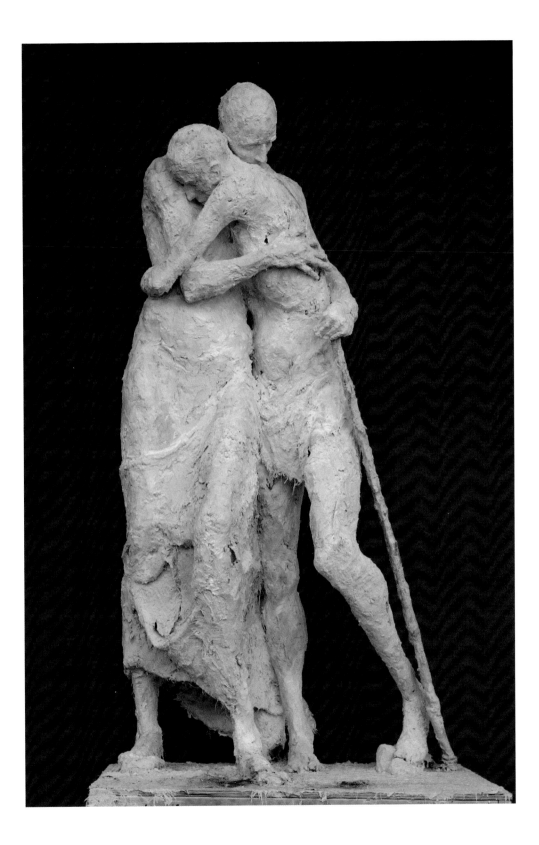

Drowning
Terra Fine
Sioux City, Iowa
Charcoal. 22" × 30". 2008.

I use charcoal to create large-scale drawings of things we see every day but rarely notice. My current drawings create a dialogue around consumption for comfort's sake, taking the viewer on an intimate journey into dietary rituals. Every day we choose to swallow things based on the reward we believe will be received (e.g., more energy, longer life, vitality, tranquility, happiness, mental focus, comfort). By choosing to draw these instances, to freeze time and enlarge the subjects, I create the opportunity for reflection about what we absent-mindedly consume day to day and what we actually gain from it.

Addiction is made up of these tiny moments, a multitude of unconscious decisions. In the life of the addicted, it is not the substance that is so appealing but the desired result, the promise of becoming the person you want to be through these substances. Focus is not placed on the act of consumption itself. If we become conscious of the taking, the consumption, to have the ability to consider and question the action, maybe we can come to grips with the addiction itself. This awareness is what is needed to begin addiction recovery.

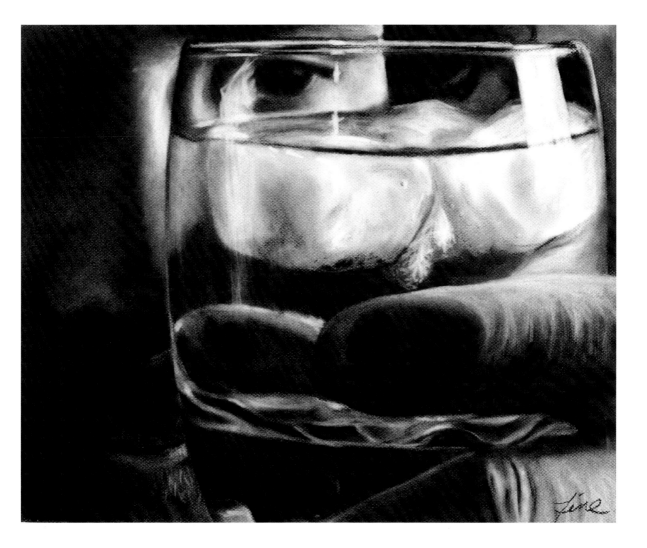

Heartache
Scott G. Brooks
Washington, D.C.
Oil on Canvas. 16" × 20". 2004.

My art portrays both the illusions of glamor and the harsh reality of abuse and addiction. Loss of control and sadness are recurring themes in my art.

My father committed suicide at age 48 after struggling with depression and addiction. Witnessing the impact his disease had on our family made an indelible impression on me. Despite this, I have alternated between anxiety about following in his footsteps and gratitude for learning from his mistakes. After years of hard work, I have moved past the fear of ending up like my father, but I must remain diligent. I am continually reminded of the links between creativity, depression, and addiction as I meet and hear the stories of other artists.

In *Heartache*, the protruding parasitic twin is the personification of addiction. She symbolizes the burden of the disease as well as the illusion of camaraderie.

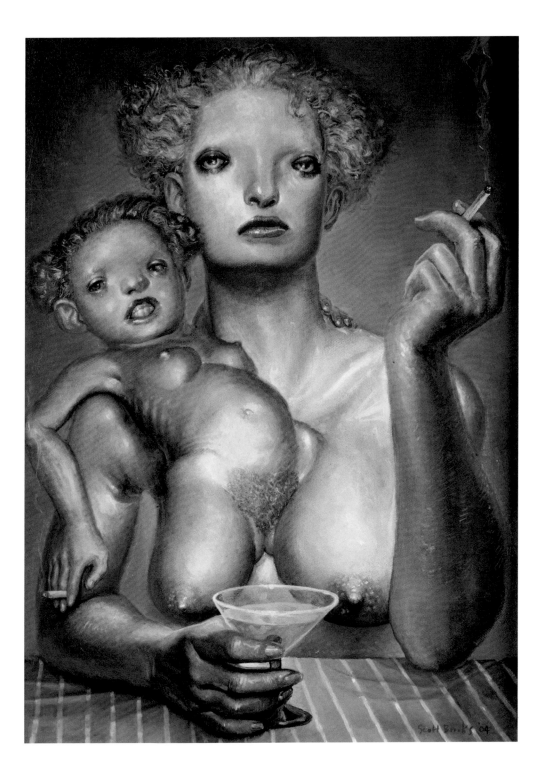

The Annunciation
Deborah Feller
New York, New York

Charcoal, White Chalk Pencils on Sepia Paper.
22" × 36". 2004.

Over the years, in my work as an addiction counselor and psychotherapist, I have been privileged to bear witness to my clients' traumatic histories and the pain accompanying their stories. Sometimes a story leaves me with an image, inspiring my next narrative work. When I have shared these ideas with my clients, they have been excited by the prospect. Together we select the particulars: props, models, setting. Later, I share preliminary sketches and, upon completion, give them an 8" × 10" signed photograph of the work.

The Annunciation shows a teenage girl and her sexual predator—her mother's boyfriend. The girl began shooting heroin and speed in her teens but now has a Ph.D. and an important role in helping children. This teen and the boy in *Toy Soldier* continue to exist unseen in the adults they have become. My drawings reveal what is rendered invisible by these inspiring recoveries.

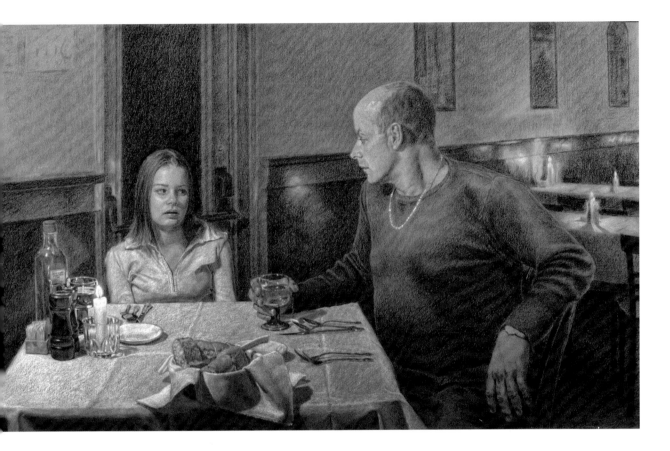

Untitled 101
Bricelyn H. Strauch
Baltimore, Maryland
Pastel. 36" × 48". 2007.

Untitled 101 explores not only the visual effects of alcohol abuse but the monotony and desperation of addiction, as well. My manipulation of the medium (pastel) and the figure through repetition, exaggerated perspective, and color composition frame substance abuse as both a physically and mentally debilitating state. This piece is meant to evoke emotions associated with isolation and introspection in the viewer, because addiction is an internal struggle, regardless of the addict's desire to quit. Addiction is a complex disease, living somewhere in the "gray" and housing many of life's enduring dichotomies (e.g., good and evil, right and wrong, lost and found). *Untitled 101* attempts to illustrate many of the contradictions that are exaggerated in the addict.

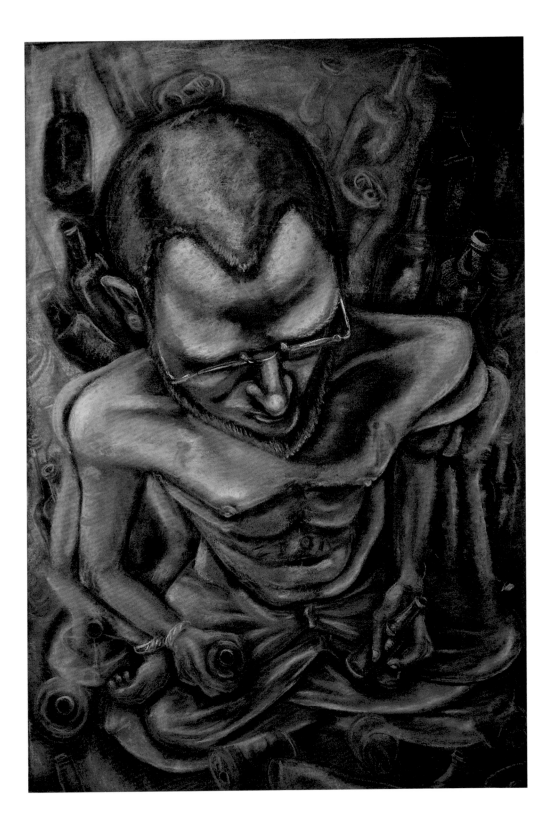

Neonate Alcoholism
Amanda Alders
Tallahassee, Florida
Acrylic on Canvas. 24" × 36". 2008.

My interest in creating *Neonate Alcoholism* was to demonstrate that addiction isn't always a choice. As an artist and a woman, I find this to be a powerful concept. Momentary decisions to indulge in a substance can have life-long consequences for the mother as well as for the unborn child. Predispositions to addiction and birth defects impact the entire family and can make recovery even more difficult. Guilt and the stress of knowing that a birth defect could have been prevented can easily lead one to continue abusing alcohol as a means of escape. While viewing the painting *Neonate Alcoholism*, I think of recovery as being an end to the cycle of generational addiction as well as being an opportunity for family members to establish a harmonious and loving home that welcomes the newborn into a world with countless possibilities.

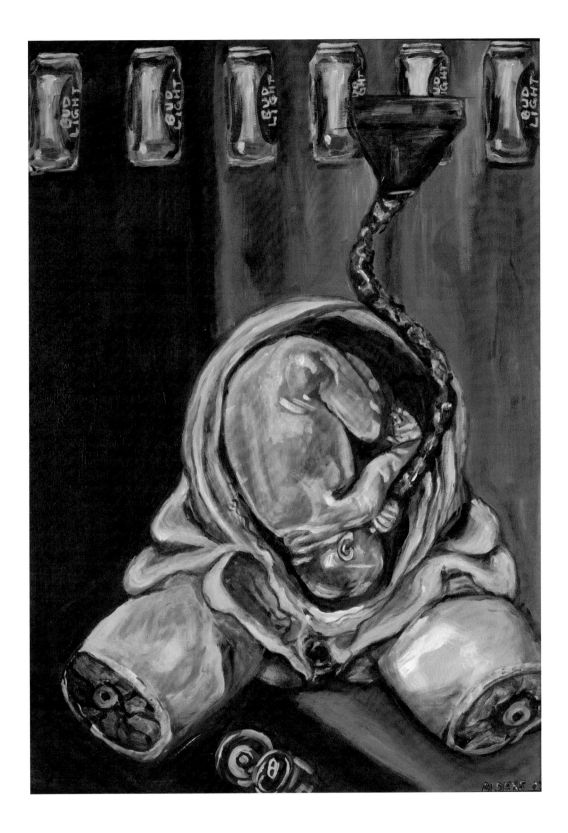

[107]

Split
Stephanie Funk
Marietta, Georgia
Watercolor, Prismacolor Markers, Ink. 7" × 8". 2008.

Having suffered the loss of friends and estrangement from family members due to alcoholism, I understand that one does not have to use substances to suffer from abuse and addiction.

In *Split*, I wanted to create a colorful atmosphere stained with black splotches that conceal alcoholic beverages. If one looks past these distracting bold spots, however, an intricate and beautiful person can be seen struggling to stay free of addiction.

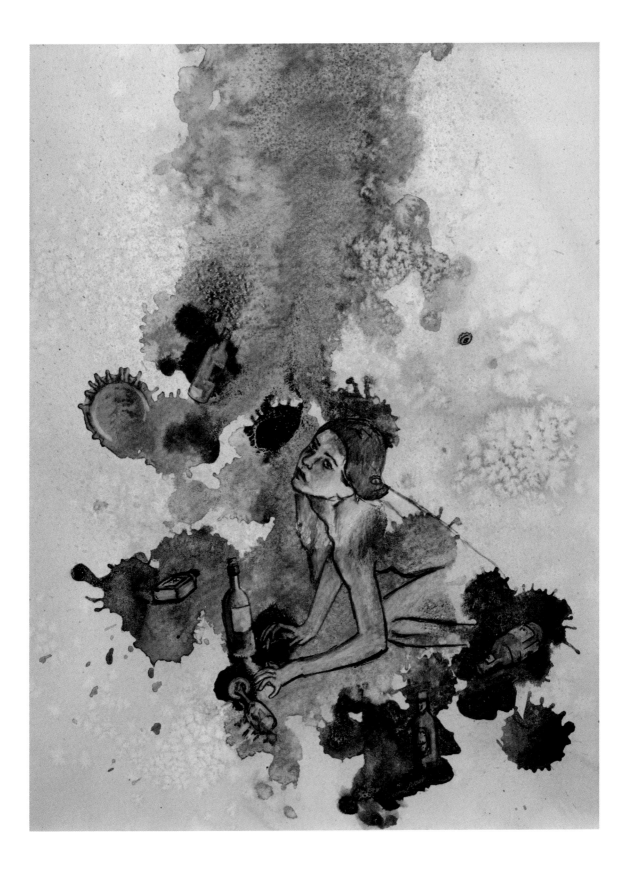

My Pill Girl
Jamie Fales
East Islip, New York

Ink, Watercolor, Colored Pencil, Graphite on Paper.
8" × 10". 2008.

I used to believe that, to produce art of any value, I had to be on pills, preferably Vicodin. It took years for me to get over that association. I realized it wasn't about the work but about my problems and numbing myself because it always seemed too hard to feel.

Art is therapeutic for me. I will work for hours on painting into the night, not realizing I missed dinner and should probably go to bed. Any piece I make has some value, even if just to me—no matter how silly, sad, serious, or sick—because it all has a part of me in it. What I blamed for my addiction has become a way of feeling and, even more so, a way of healing for me.

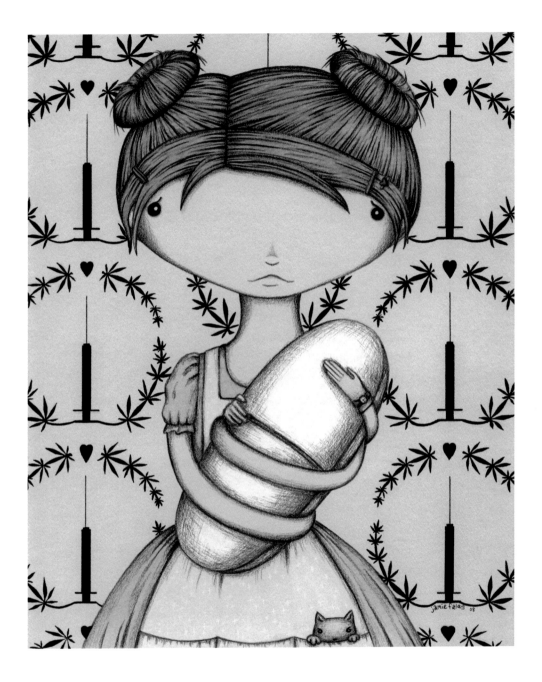

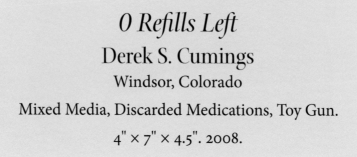

0 Refills Left
Derek S. Cumings
Windsor, Colorado
Mixed Media, Discarded Medications, Toy Gun.
4" × 7" × 4.5". 2008.

From conception I knew this piece would spark questions in everyone, based on his or her own personal experiences—signifying either a long, drawn-out battle or the instantaneous loss of someone you love. Someone, without too much notice, has slipped from a once strong grasp of reality. Some will not see the juxtaposition if they only see medication as a tool of help. I hope most see medication as the double-edged sword it has become. Why don't we secure medicine cabinets half as well as gun cabinets?

Using an old toy gun and approximately 550–600 discarded prescription pills, I have attempted to not only open eyes but also open a small door into my life. Five years ago, I suffered a short fall that left two discs in my back in disrepair, ending my active life as I had known it. The combination of muscle relaxers, opiates, anti-nausea drugs, sleep aids, mood stabilizers, and antidepressants may help make the day-to-day tolerable, but these medications also work against my artist drive, which was once strongest in my 18th or 19th hour of the day.

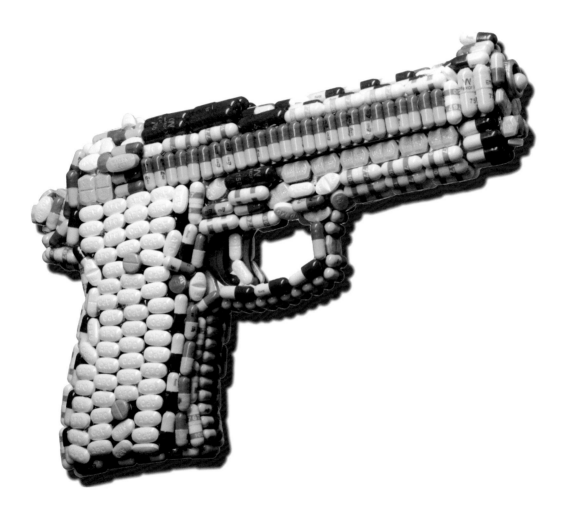

Untitled, I
John Bierner
Fajardo, Puerto Rico
Oil Paint. 20" × 27". 2002.

I've been affected by heroin and other drugs since I was a child. One of my favorite uncles (now in prison because of drug addiction) introduced me to some of the harder drugs when I was a teenager. I would smoke PCP and use coke with him. I haven't used heroin in over 10 years. Many of my family members ended up being "junkies" and "crack heads." Heroin has always been a major issue in my family.

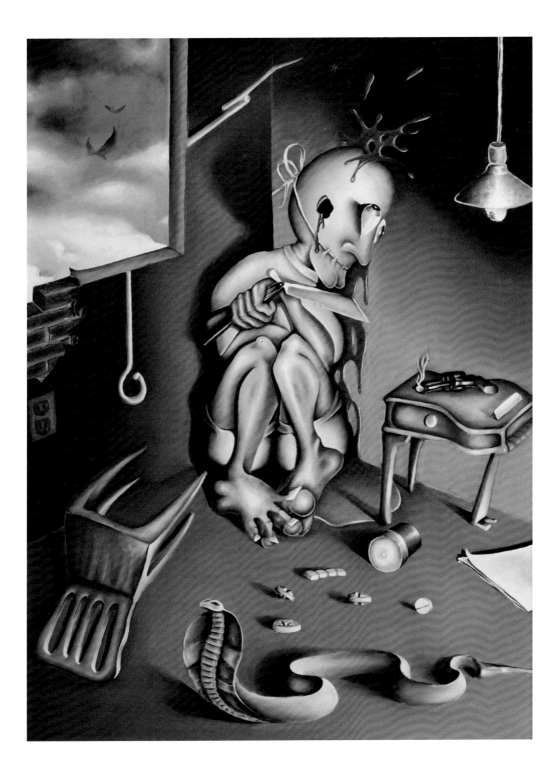

Allegory of Abundance and Denial
Andrew Cooper

Cardiff, Wales, United Kingdom

Sculpture, Photograph. 6' × 3'. 2006.

The title references a drawing by Botticelli and paintings by Bruegel and van Savoy in which the cornucopia overflows, symbolizing the allegorical figures of Peace, Luck, and Concord. The horn of plenty has the power to continuously refill itself with everything its owner might desire, to bestow contentment or harmony. My vision of the relationship between desire, providence, and plenty is one in which the cornucopia spews out its contents, cradling the addict who can feel whole and human only in its morbid embrace; the downward spiral through craving and obsession, reducing him to a solitary and jaundiced figure, seemingly hovering close to death.

The chiaroscuro-lit figure appears as if in the late stages of uncontrollable addiction, bereft and unconcerned for all other comforts. The only essential is the "fix." This solitary figure is yellowed and bruised and appears to float in mid-air. He has soiled himself, suggesting a semi-comatose state in which bodily functions have begun to shut down in the final throes of drug dependency.

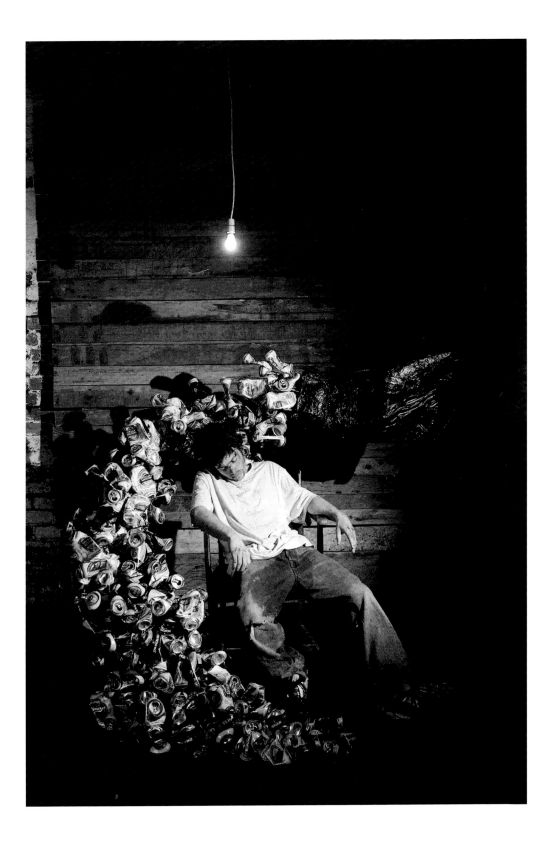

Driving under the Influence
Linda Ruiz
Palmdale, California

Photograph. 11" × 14". 2008.

Driving under the influence is no laughing matter and should not be taken lightly. *Driving under the Influence* is a caricature of someone who has taken one too many.

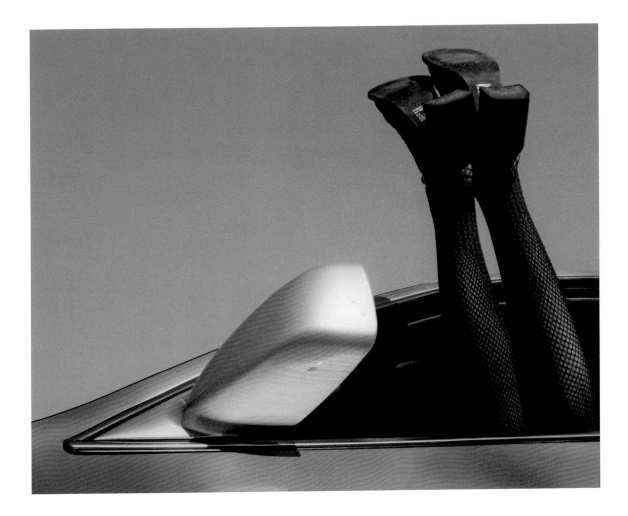

Recovery 3
Tom Hill
Brentwood, Maryland
Computer-generated Image. 7.5" × 10". 2008.

I combine words and written material with visual images as printed matter that takes the form of page design, posters and flyers, and books. Blending the personal and the political, my work conveys my experience in the world as a gay man in recovery from addiction. I seek to create art that can serve as a catalyst of an inward-outward journey, satisfying my need for spiritual exploration and healing, and to communicate an activism focused on social justice and human liberation. I use computer-generated images in a way that evokes the intimacy of personal journaling to stimulate thought and dialogue and to pack the punch of agitation and propaganda.

I am in recovery from addiction. Becoming addicted to substances and behaviors was not my fault. Addiction was not the result of bad choices. The most important choice I made was a positive one. I decided I wanted to be in recovery. Today, my main responsibility is to nurture and maintain my recovery. Practicing a daily routine to build spiritual muscle, I try to be useful and be of service to others. In this way, I am able to give back and replace the things I took during my addiction. Most of all, I want my recovery to be a light to shine for those who are still living in the darkness of addiction. I am in recovery from addiction. Becoming addicted to substances and behaviors was not my fault. Addiction was not the result of bad choices. The most important choice I made was a positive one. I decided I wanted to be in recovery. Today, my main responsibility is to nurture and maintain my recovery. Practicing a daily routine to build spiritual muscle, I try to be useful and be of service to others. In this way, I am able to give back and replace the things I took during my addiction. Most of all, I want my recovery to be a light to shine for those who are still living in the darkness of addiction.

Tom Hill 2008

Angst
Ralph Irby
Norfolk, Virginia
Charcoal. 22" × 28". 2007.

I retired in 2005 from my job as a Norfolk Master Police Officer with over 25 years of service. The majority of my career I served as an investigator assigned to the Vice and Narcotics Division. I have worked numerous undercover assignments and joint narcotics task forces throughout Hampton Roads. I have received numerous letters of commendation from the Drug Enforcement Administration, the Federal Bureau of Investigation, and local law enforcement agencies, civic groups, and charitable organizations.

Speaking about drug awareness to the youth of my community is one of my greatest joys. I decided to attend Old Dominion University after I retired to pursue my Master of Fine Arts degree. Exhibiting my artwork during these talks is a big part of my message. I have always had a passion for drawing; I find it to be an excellent vehicle for dialogue. I find it most rewarding to incorporate my life experiences with my passion for drawing. How does this relate to drug addiction and recovery? As a retired narcotics investigator and an artist, I personally believe that empathic listening can promote mutual healing and mutual understanding of the most painful conflicts.

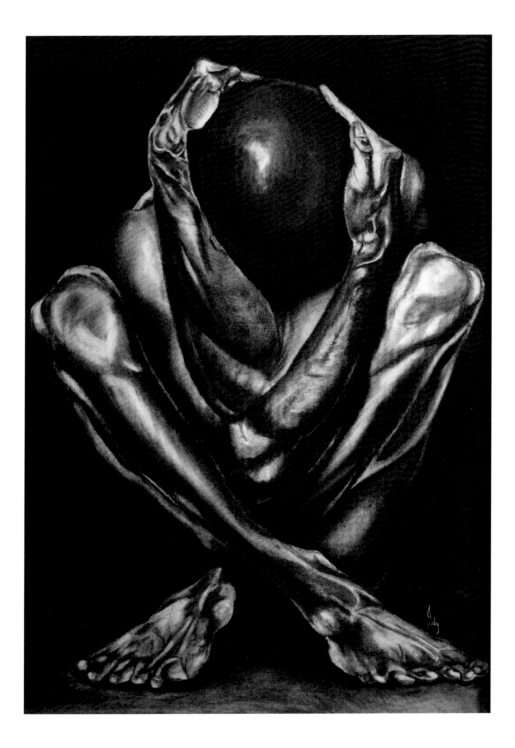

Get Humble Now
Parker W. Lanier
Holland, Michigan
Markers. 19" × 19". 2008.

When I got out of rehab in February 2002, I had to change everything I did if I wanted to stay sober. This included not only going to a lot of AA meetings but doing things that would occupy the time I would have spent drinking.

I saw some people journaling, so I started drawing. I started filling sketch books... Art is one of the ways I am carrying the message of recovery.

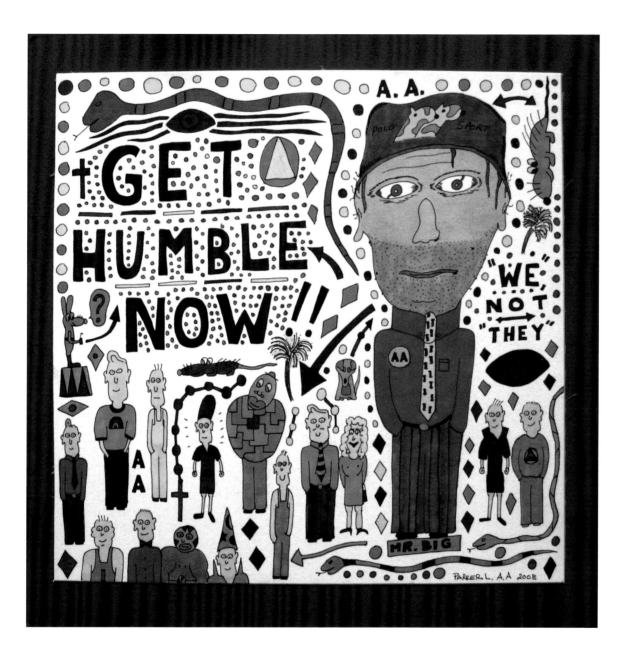

Ask Again Tomorrow...
Lindsey Mears
Charlottesville, Virginia

Mixed Media. 32" × 23". 2008.

Ask Again Tomorrow... is my visual representation of the dichotomy of addiction as I have experienced it—allure and shame. It is about the "push-pull" of being lifted into a state of perceived love, communion, and grace alternating with the weight of all the strings left untied—the real interactions avoided, real wishes thwarted, energy displaced and wasted.

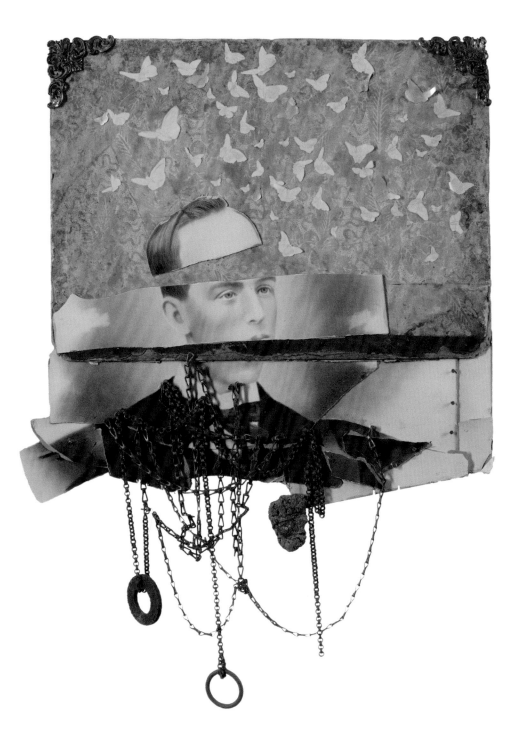

Hands of Recovery
Sam T. Barnes
Cookeville, Tennessee
Bronze Sculpture. 12" × 12" × 12". 2007.

We admitted we were powerless over alcohol—that our lives had become unmanageable.

Step One of the Twelve Steps of Alcoholics Anonymous

Practicing orthopedic surgery supports my sculpting materially; whereas sculpting is one of the mainstays of my spiritual life. The power of a spiritual life began to dawn on me 9 years ago when I began working the 12 steps of recovery. Attempting to portray these steps by the expression of bronze sculptures of hands has helped me tremendously in my growth. I find that the hard work and sometimes the mystery of the foundry—a process I refer to as "art-reco" (short for art recovery)—supplies me with the balance my life needs.

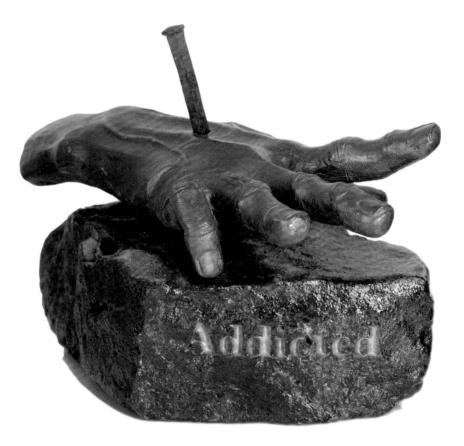

Sometimes It's the Small Things
Jim Bycznski
Berea, Ohio
Acrylic on Canvas. 24" × 32". 2007.

I learned first-hand how addiction can put a strangle-hold on those you love. My father loved us but was too weak to break free from the allure of his dependency. My father was an alcoholic, as was his father before him. I could have followed the same path. It would have been easy. I saw the possibilities of my lineage while in college. I experienced how easy it is to fall, how one drink turns to two, two into three, etc. How it progresses from social situations to everyday routines.

My children are my strength. They are the light that keeps me from the path of darkness. This painting is a reflection of how sometimes it's the small things that cause us to pause, to re-evaluate our direction and break the cycle. The young life reaches out to its mother as if to say, "STOP! I will be your reason to quit. I will be there to help mend your soul, while giving you strength to move forward with your life."

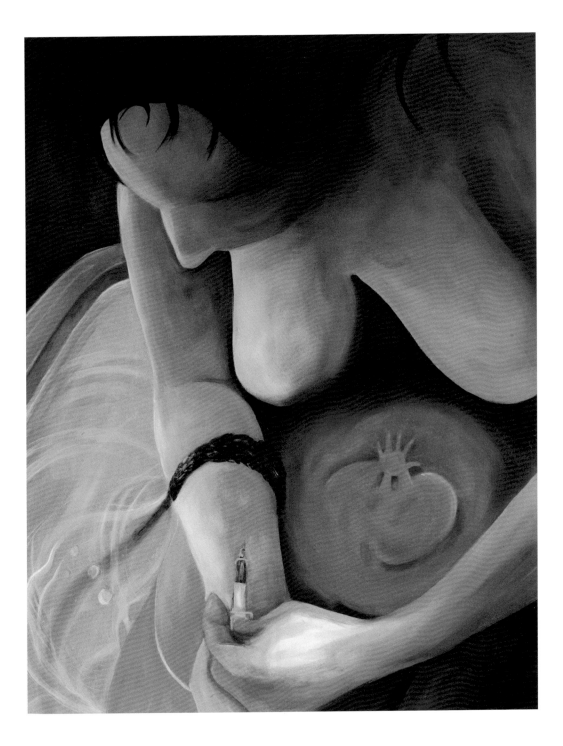

Couple
Sam Fuchs and Adam Gray
Burlingame, California
Digital Inkjet Print. 32" × 40". 2007.

The signature characteristic of our work is the use of thousands of miniature icons compiled together to create a single object. The contrast in dimensions of the icons and the master object invite the viewer to dive deeper into the image, to see irony and hypocrisy revealed. Drug abuse, subcultures, capitalism, art snobbery, and hyped-up fads stand out as themes in our convoluted compositions. Our work can be considered extreme Pop art, a social commentary often focusing on the neo-kitsch trademarks of today's hipster culture: party, sleaze, and current affairs.

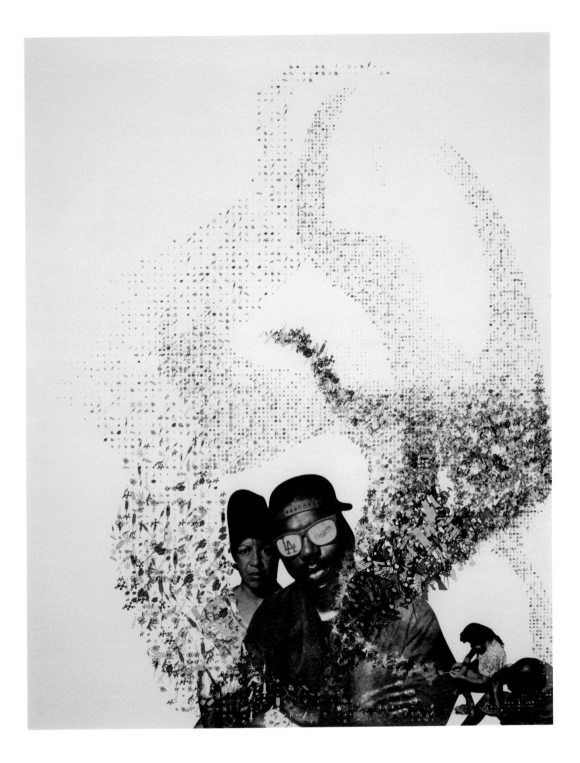

After Richter
Christina Z. Anderson
Bozeman, Montana
Gelatin Silver Mordançage. 11" × 14". 2003.

I am the parent of an addict—an adult child addicted to drugs, then food (bulimia), then alcohol. To watch the downward spiral over the last 13 years has been the most difficult experience of my life. There was hope this year: she entered treatment for a period of 3.5 months. She has, however, returned to alcohol. As a parent, I have had to detach and draw boundaries to remain stable. I am blessed to be able to work through some of the grief through my photography.

After Richter, depicting a disintegrating person, is representative of addiction. The print is a black-and-white photograph that has been subjected to an intense chemical acid bath that disintegrates the dark portions proportionately to the amount of silver present. This process, known as mordançage, is a fitting one to describe the process of addiction, as both take a whole object or person and destroy through chemical means.

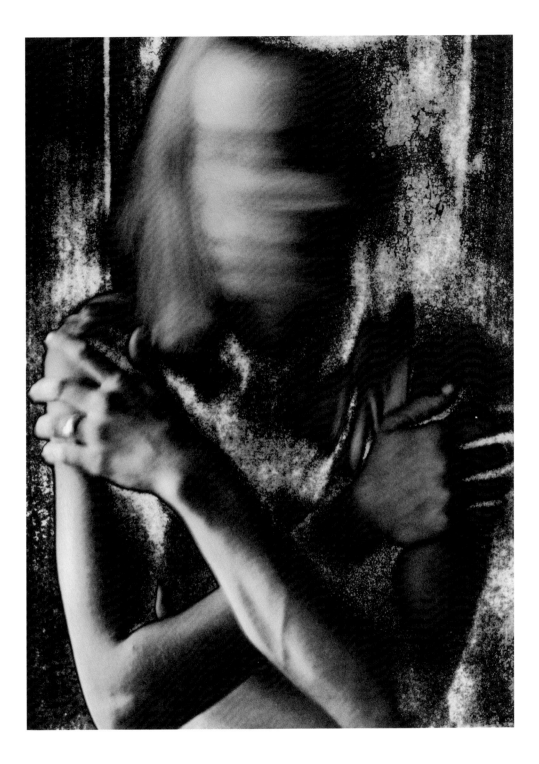

Restoration of the Spirit
Maryellen Cox
Bargersville, Indiana
Ink, Acrylic, and Plaster on Board. 17" × 22.5". 2004.

Smoking was part of my family for as long as I could remember. My father and his eight siblings smoked; all of them suffered from emphysema. My brother died of lung cancer. I knew I would be okay; I could stop smoking at any time. Things began to change in my life. My son had had respiratory problems since infancy. My hand always held a cigarette. My laugh turned into a wheeze. It was time.

Restoration of a painting requires patience and time. Repairing fragment damage to the foundation enhances a painting's overall strength and beauty. Conquering my smoking addiction also required patience, time, and acceptance of self. In the process of repairing my own spirit and body by giving up the dependence, I found new depth within myself. I became an artist and a teacher. This enhanced strength extended not only to my family but to those whose lives I touch. Putting out that last cigarette was my new beginning.

Restoration of the Spirit was created to reflect hope and emergence from a damaged spirit and being. The parts that still adhere to the foundation reveal what comprised the original.

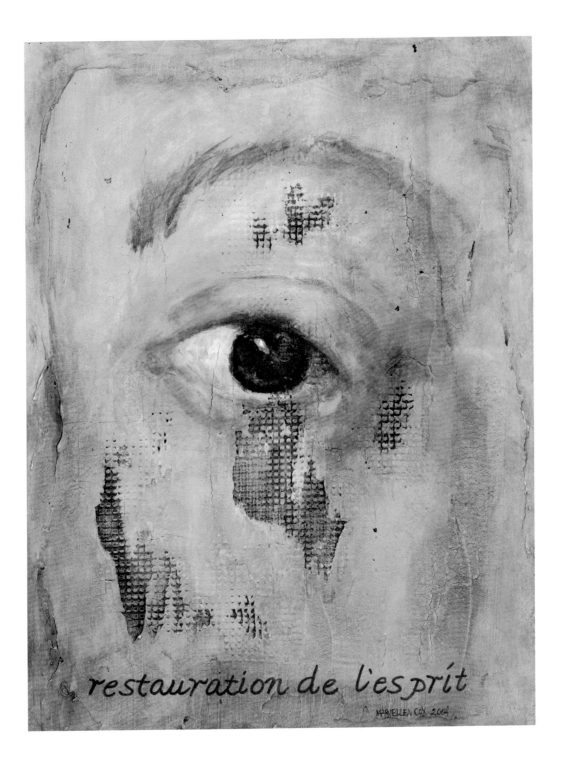

restauration de l'esprit

MARIELLEN COX 2004

Epilogue

The art presented in this book reveals the complex struggles of individuals entrapped in a life ruled by drug addiction. Several books and articles—including our own[1]—address the science of addiction, but few address addiction from the perspective of artists. Art can complement science in developing a thorough understanding of the human dimensions of addiction and recovery. Talented visual artists have provided unique insights through their art as they capture both the destructive power of addiction and the new life born in recovery.

From nearly 1,000 images submitted for possible publication in this book, we attempted to find some balance among the various themes and perspectives. These included the telling of authentic addiction stories through the art, striving to achieve the goal of maintaining the artistic and intellectual honesty of the collection, and, finally, addressing the sensibilities of those who journey through this book. These strategies directed our efforts in support of the primary goal of using this collection to reveal the human experience of addiction and recovery to allow readers to reach a new understanding of addiction—perhaps an understanding that connected with their own ideas and that may have been informed through their own experiences and those of friends and loved ones.

Through these images, we hope readers will better understand the experience of addiction and, in the process, reclaim a human connection with individuals who suffer from this treatable medical illness. The collection provides opportunities to help change awareness, broaden understanding, and alter our behavior. By inviting us to engage with the experience of addiction and recovery in an immediate and personal way, art helps us move beyond stigma and stereotypes to recognize that substance abuse and addiction are *our* problem as a community, not just *their* failing as individuals.

As important as it is to explain what we hoped to accomplish and the strategies we used, it is also important to explain what we were not attempting. This book is not intended to prevent or treat addiction, and the art was not selected with the goal of using it in antidrug posters or campaigns, although we believe that some of it does have that potential. In fact, not all of the art paints the horrendous picture of addiction which might serve to powerfully dissuade people from using drugs. We hope that the images will not stir longings to resume drug use in those struggling to maintain their freedom from abuse and addiction, but we did not reject images simply because of such concerns. Indeed, we recognize that such triggers are ubiquitous and range from the smell of money to advertisements for tobacco and alcohol to the places an individual associates with addiction. We do hope that even people facing such struggles may find insights in this book which will strengthen their efforts to seek and maintain drug-free lives, even if some images are difficult for them to view.

Epilogue

One of the concerns discussed by our advisory board was whether some images in this book would contain triggers that might provoke relapse among individuals in recovery. In fact, extensive research has been conducted on the relationship between types of situations that can trigger or precipitate relapse to alcohol, tobacco, or other drug use.[2] Addiction scientists have examined several factors leading to relapse and have compiled a virtual taxonomy, or list, of relapse triggers. These include exposure to drug-related cues (seeing the drug, being offered the drug, associating with other drug users), experiencing various emotional states (feelings of boredom, anger, frustration, worry, anxiety, sadness, etc.), and coping with high-risk situations. Addiction scientists have organized factors that trigger relapse into specific inventories of drinking or drug-taking situations for the purpose of developing useful treatment interventions to prevent relapse.[3] Part of the goal is to help those in recovery achieve and sustain drug abstinence by learning to manage their responses to stimuli that could trigger drug use. While this book is not intended to be part of addiction treatment programs, we hope that some recovering individuals will find it useful in their efforts to achieve freedom from drugs through insight drawn from the images presented.

Although the focus is on the visual art, the words of the artists are intended to help in understanding the art itself and addiction more broadly. Many have told us that they gain the greatest insights by viewing the art first without reading the artist's statement, then reading the statement, and then reexamining the art. Through their art and accompanying statements, the artists described wrenching addiction experiences in phrases like these: "I suffered"..."I was chained"..."my total despair"..."I struggled"..."sometimes I had hope ... less often I had help"..."cruel bondage"..."I broke free"..."I found my voice through art"..."I live again." Hearing these descriptions of addiction and experiencing the art unleashed emotional responses in our advisory group which were stunning to comprehend. Some of the art can be disturbing, confusing, challenging, even repulsive. The images might elicit feelings of sorrow, anger, or despair; might frighten or seduce. To answer the question raised in the introduction—"What does art have to do with addiction?"—the collection embodies one master story: substance abuse and addiction are not, and have never been, simple phenomena to understand, treat, or prevent.

The art has inspired us to offer different strategies to educate and prevent substance abuse and addiction using our model of addiction art exhibitions. Based on our experience of the past five years, these exhibitions have struck a vital and responsive chord among members of our neighborhood communities as well as professionals working in the substance abuse field. The collection gives us the inspiration and drive to make a difference in reducing addiction and helping people achieve recovery. We trust that readers will also be inspired by the art to ask, in the words of former Surgeon General C. Everett Koop, "What can I do to help fight addiction instead of fighting those who have it?"

The addiction art displayed in this book strives to offer insight, guidance, and hope based on noteworthy points of consensus. Several key consensus points have emerged, underscoring the pivotal role that addiction art plays in the education and prevention of substance use disorders.

First, addiction art can contribute to changing the way individuals understand substance use disorders (abuse and addiction), from seeing them as a weakness or a moral failing deserving of punishment to accepting them as chronic medical illnesses requiring treatment. Understanding addiction as a treatable medical illness is essential in preventing and reducing this prevalent public health problem. Second, the educational component of addiction art complements addiction science. Addiction art exhibitions, such as those that led to this book, present riveting personal stories and stamp lasting images on audiences of all ages. Learning that addiction is a medical illness touching all aspects of humanity will lead to the kind of compassion and understanding that can contribute to prevention and treatment. Third, addiction science can benefit from the visual arts, which can draw attention to our country's unmet need for available and accessible addiction treatment, prevention, and education to control and reduce substance use disorders. Finally, addiction art exhibitions can range from those drawn from national and international domains to those emerging from neighborhood communities, and despite diverse origins, such art can live and work well together.

Addiction art communicates at a more basic level than that of the intellectual demand for facts and figures. It teaches its lessons through primal emotional reactions, which can stand alone, and perhaps in some cases reinforces or even challenges facts and figures. Addiction art should not be viewed as secondary to the transmission of factual information; fact and art are equally important in understanding addiction.

Finally, we hope that the art and stories presented in this book will help to inspire:

- in family and friends, the compassion that can drive the often challenging struggle to support the efforts of loved ones to achieve freedom from addiction;
- in those ruled by addiction, the knowledge that recovery is attainable and that they are not alone in their struggle;
- in policymakers, the will to provide adequate funding for addiction

treatment and prevention at the federal, state, and community levels to
help those afflicted; and

- in addiction scientists, a better understanding of the human dimensions of this treatable medical illness they are investigating.

If this book contributes in any small way to meet these aspirations, then we
will have achieved our goal.

APPENDIX A

Addiction Art Advisory Board

Innovators Combating Substance Abuse
National Program Office
Department of Psychiatry and Behavioral Sciences
The Johns Hopkins University School of Medicine

ANITA BOLES, M.P.A., Executive Director, Society for the Arts in Healthcare, Washington, DC

PETER BRUUN, Artist/Director, Art on Purpose, Baltimore, MD

F. LENNOX CAMPELLO, Director, Daily Campello Art News, Potomac, MD

PATRICK COGGINS, Ph.D., Professor, Stetson University, DeLand, FL

BETTE-JANE CRIGGER, Ph.D., Director, Ethics Policy, and Secretary, Council on Ethical and Judicial Affairs, American Medical Association, Chicago, IL

MARGARET L. DOWELL, Ph.D., Artist and Adjunct Professor, Mount St. Mary's University, Emmitsburg, MD, and Carroll Community College, Westminster, MD

LILLIAN FITZGERALD, Founder and Director, Fitzgerald Fine Art, and Curator, Clinical Research Center Art Program, National Institutes of Health, Bethesda, MD

JACK E. HENNINGFIELD, Ph.D., Director, Robert Wood Johnson Foundation's Innovators Combating Substance Abuse, National Program Office at the Johns Hopkins University School of Medicine, Professor, Behavioral Biology at the Johns Hopkins University School of Medicine, and Vice President, Research and Health Policy, Pinney Associates, Bethesda, MD

TRAVIS HENNINGFIELD, College Student, the Pratt Institute, Brooklyn, NY

TERRANCE KEENAN, M.L.S., Artist and Author, Monkton, MD

C. EVERETT KOOP, M.D., Sc.D., Senior Scholar, the C. Everett Koop Institute at Dartmouth, the Elizabeth DeCamp McInerny Professor of Surgery, Dartmouth Medical School, Hanover, NH, and U.S. Surgeon General (1981–1989)

FRED LAZARUS, IV, President, the Maryland Institute College of Art, Baltimore, MD

DENNIS O. ROMERO, Deputy Center Director, Center for Substance Abuse Prevention, Substance Abuse and Mental Health Services Administration, Rockville, MD

PATRICIA B. SANTORA, Ph.D., Deputy Director, Robert Wood Johnson Foundation's Innovators Combating Substance Abuse, National Program Office at the Johns Hopkins University School of Medicine, and Assistant Professor, Psychiatry, the Johns Hopkins University School of Medicine

ED SINGLETON, Ph.D., Senior Clinical Associate, Center for Prevention and Treatment Research, the Maya Tech Corporation, Silver Spring, MD

DENNIS TARTAGLIA, President, Tartaglia Communications, Somerset, NJ

KIMA J. TAYLOR, M.D., Director, Drug Addiction Treatment Program, Open Society Institute, Baltimore, MD

SHARON WALSH, Ph.D., Director, Center on Drug and Alcohol Research, University of Kentucky College of Medicine, Lexington, KY, President, College on Problems of Drug Dependence (2008/2009)

MARK H. WARD, Deputy Director, the American Visionary Art Museum, Baltimore, MD

"Call to Artists": Method of Gathering Art for This Collection

Our national "Call to Artists" (reproduced below) was widely circulated through print and electronic media to reach a broad audience of artists. The call provided artists with a four-month period (November 2007 through February 2008) to create a new work of art on our theme of addiction and recovery. We placed the notice in a variety of art journals, magazines, and websites, including *American Artist*, *Art Calendar*, *Art Deadlines*, *Art in America*, *College Art Association*, *Daily Campello Art News* (formerly *Mid-Atlantic Art News*), and the *Society for the Arts in Healthcare*. We also distributed it at alcohol and drug treatment and prevention centers and at professional substance abuse and art therapy conferences.

The call was mailed to all 86 art colleges in the United States, and administrators at each of these colleges were personally contacted with a request to post the notice on school bulletin boards to attract faculty and student interest. The call was also mailed to all artists who had submitted art for the Innovators Program's previous addiction art exhibitions. In addition, numerous presentations and contacts were made with local art leagues, art galleries, and artists about submitting entries to be judged and selected for this collection.

CALL TO ARTISTS

Putting a Human Face on Addiction and Recovery

Deadline for Submissions: March 1, 2008

Sponsored by:
Innovators Combating Substance Abuse Program
at The Johns Hopkins University School of Medicine
http://www.innovatorsawards.org

Supported by:
The Robert Wood Johnson Foundation
http://www.rwjf.org

CALL TO ARTISTS

ART AND ADDICTION

Dear Artist,

The **Innovators Combating Substance Abuse Program** is pleased to issue a *Call to Artists* whose original art will be selected to appear in a book on art and addiction that is being considered for publication by the Johns Hopkins University Press. The Innovators Program, supported by The Robert Wood Johnson Foundation, is a national program based in the Department of Psychiatry and Behavioral Sciences at the Johns Hopkins University School of Medicine in Baltimore.

The purpose of the proposed book is to provide a stimulus to change the way America views addiction by using the visual arts to put a human face on addiction and recovery. Creativity and artistic expression play a significant role both in recovery and in raising awareness of the personal toll caused by substance abuse and addiction. The proposed book on addiction art is intended to complement and serve as the companion volume to the editors' book on addiction science, *Addiction Treatment: Science and Policy for the Twenty-First Century* (JE Henningfield, PB Santora, WK Bickel (eds), Johns Hopkins Press, November 2007).

We invite all artists to submit original artwork on the theme of drug addiction and recovery (drugs include alcohol, tobacco, illegal, or prescription drugs). A distinguished panel of jurors, composed of prominent members from both the art and addiction science communities, will select the art for the book. Finalists will receive an honorarium of $200, with the top five finalists receiving an additional honorarium of $500; a copy of the book, and will be included in exhibitions in Maryland (May 2008) and at the annual meeting of the College on Problems of Drug Dependence in Puerto Rico (June 14-19, 2008). Other exhibition possibilities are pending at this time.

Works submitted may be in any media, including video. Works included in the book will not be limited to size, but extreme size may limit works for inclusion in the exhibitions.

Attached are the submission guidelines and a submission form. For additional information, please contact the Innovators Program at (443) 287-3915 or visit our website (www.innovatorsawards.org).

We strongly believe that art can help bridge the gap between addiction science and the human experience of addition. Thank you for your interest and for providing insight that science cannot match.

Appendix B

Authors
Patricia B. Santora, PhD
Deputy Director, Innovators National Program Office
Assistant Professor, Department of Psychiatry and Behavioral Sciences, the Johns
      Hopkins University School of Medicine

Margaret Dowell, PhD
Artist and Professor, Adjunct, Department of Education, Mount Saint Mary's University

Jack E. Henningfield, PhD
Director, Innovators National Program Office
Professor, Adjunct, Department of Psychiatry and Behavioral Sciences, the Johns
      Hopkins University School of Medicine

SUBMISSION GUIDELINES

The book's theme is Drug Addiction and Recovery. The content of artwork should be a narrative of, reflection upon, or expression about some aspect of this theme. Jurors are particularly interested in seeing the human side of addiction and recovery. Artworks will be judged based upon how effectively, clearly, and expressively the book's theme is explored.

THE FOLLOWING GUIDELINES APPLY TO ALL SUBMISSIONS:

Eligibility:
    Works in all media including video will be accepted.
    Works may be any size.
    Works may have been completed in any year.

Entry:
    Artists may submit up to 3 artworks in slide or digital format.

    For Slides: Label each slide with your name and title of work on the front of the slide. Please indicate the top of the slide. Place slides in an "8 ½ x 11" clear vinyl slide sheet holder. Write your name on the holder.
    For CDs: Label each file with your name and title of work. Write your name on the CD holder. Submit images in .jpeg format, resolution 72dpi; file size should not exceed 1mb.
    For Digital Images Submitted by E-Mail: Label each image with your name and title of work. Submit images in .jpeg format, resolution 72dpi; file size should not exceed 1mb. Email digital submissions to: innovatorsawards@jhmi.edu.

    Artists must submit a 100-200 word Artist Statement which addresses the relationship between the artist / the work and the "Drug Addiction and Recovery" theme.

Artists must also complete and submit the Submission Form.

SEND SUBMISSIONS TO: Innovators Combating Substance Abuse Program, The Johns Hopkins University School of Medicine, 600 N. Wolfe Street, Meyer Building 3-142, Baltimore, MD 21287

For additional information, please contact the Innovators Program at (443) 287-3915 or visit our website (www.innovatorsawards.org).

Book and Exhibition Calendar:

March 1, 2008	Entry Deadline (Postmarked Date)
April 1, 2008	Notification of Acceptance
April 10, 2008	Deadline for Delivery of Accepted Artworks
May 2008	Conference Exhibition, Maryland
June 14-19, 2008	Conference Exhibition, College on Problems of Drug Dependence, San Juan, Puerto Rico
July 15, 2008	Art Work Returned (Pending no other venues for exhibits)
September 2008	Book Manuscript Submitted for Possible Publication by the Johns Hopkins Press

SUBMISSION FORM

After reviewing submission guidelines, complete the information below. Be sure to include a 100-200 word artist statement. You may submit up to 3 pieces for consideration. **Deadline for receipt of all materials is March 1, 2008.**

Name:

_____

Mailing Address:

_____

_____

E-Mail Address:

_____

Telephone Number:

_____

Website (Optional):

_____

#1 Title:
Media:
Dimensions:
Year of Completion:

#2 Title:
Media:
Dimensions:
Year of Completion:

#3 Title:
Media:
Dimensions:
Year of Completion:

CONDITIONS OF PARTICIPATION: *I understand that any damage or loss of artwork resulting from its inclusion in the Art & Addiction book and exhibitions is not the responsibility of any party involved in the book or exhibitions, including but not limited to The Innovators Combating Substance Abuse Program. As the artist and lender of the artwork, I assume all risk of damage or loss. Furthermore, if my artwork is selected, I hereby give my permission to the Innovators Combating Substance Abuse Program to publish my artwork in their book, newsletter, on their website, in their 2009 Art & Addiction calendar as well as to publicize my work through the media at no charge.*

Print Name:_____

Signature:_____Date:_____

NOTES

Introduction

1. Johnston LD, O'Malley PM, Bachman JG, Schulenberg JE. 2008. *Monitoring the Future: National Results on Adolescent Drug Use: Overview of Key Findings, 2007* (NIH Publication No. 08-6418). Bethesda, MD: National Institute on Drug Abuse.

2. The National Center on Addiction and Substance Abuse (CASA) at Columbia University. 2007. *Wasting the Best and the Brightest: Substance Abuse at America's Colleges and Universities.* New York: The National Center on Addiction and Substance Abuse (CASA) at Columbia University.

ONE: Cultivating the Visual Arts to Stimulate Insights into Addiction and Recovery

1. Centers for Disease Control and Prevention. 2004. *The Burden of Chronic Diseases and Their Risk Factors: National and State Perspectives 2004.* Atlanta: U.S. Department of Health and Human Services.

2. Santora PB, Hutton HE. 2008. Longitudinal trends in hospital admissions with co-occurring alcohol/drug diagnoses, 1994–2002. *Journal of Substance Abuse Treatment* 35: 1–12.

3. Institute of Medicine of the National Academies. 2006. *Improving the Quality of Health Care for Mental and Substance-Use Conditions: Quality Chasm Series.* Washington, DC: National Academies Press.

4. Mokdad AH, Marks JS, Stroup DF, Gerberding JL. 2004. Actual causes of death in the United States, 2000. *Journal of the American Medical Association* 291:1238–1245.

5. Morbidity and Mortality Weekly Report. 2005. Annual smoking-attributable mortality, years of potential life lost, and productivity losses, United States, 1997–2001. *Morbidity and Mortality Weekly Report* 54:625–628.

6. Mark TL, Coffey RM, McKusick DR, et al. 2005. *National Estimates of Expenditures for Mental Health Services and Substance Abuse Treatment, 1991–*

2001. Rockville, MD: Substance Abuse and Mental Health Services Administration (Publication No. SMA05-3999).

7. Office of National Drug Control Policy. 2004. *The Economic Costs of Drug Abuse in the United States, 1992–2002.* Washington, DC: Executive Office of the President (Publication No. 207303).

8. Henningfield JE, Santora PB, Bickel WK (Eds). 2007. *Addiction Treatment: Science and Policy for the Twenty-first Century.* Baltimore: Johns Hopkins University Press.

9. Koop CE. 2006. Health and health care for the 21st century: For all the people. *American Journal of Public Health* 96(12):2090–2092.

10. Koop CE. 2007. Drug addiction in America: Challenges and opportunities. In JE Henningfield, PB Santora, and WK Bickel, eds., *Addiction Treatment: Science and Policy for the Twenty-first Century.* Baltimore: Johns Hopkins University Press.

11. Henningfield, Santora, Bickel, 2007.

12. Leshner AI. 2007. Advancing the science base for the treatment of addiction. In JE Henningfield, PB Santora, and WK Bickel, eds., *Addiction Treatment: Science and Policy for the Twenty-first Century.* Baltimore: Johns Hopkins University Press.

13. Miller WR, Carroll KM (Eds). 2006. *Rethinking Substance Abuse: What the Science Shows, and What We Should Do about It.* New York: The Guilford Press.

14. Koop CE. 2003. Drug addiction in America: Challenges and opportunities (special feature). *Military Medicine* 168:viii–xvi.

15. McLellan AT. 2006. What we need is a system: Creating a responsive and effective substance abuse treatment system. In WR Miller and KM Carroll, eds., *Rethinking Substance Abuse: What the Science Shows, and What We Should Do about It.* New York: The Guilford Press.

16. Leshner, 2007.

17. Isaacs SL, Knickman JR (Eds). 2006. *To Improve Health and Health Care, Volume X.* San Francisco: Jossey-Bass.

18. Institute of Medicine, 2006.

19. Miller, Carroll, 2006.

20. Shilts R. 1987. *And the Band Played On: Politics, People and the AIDS Epidemic.* New York: St. Martin's Press.

21. Kushner T. 1993/1994. *Angels in America: A Gay Fantasia on National Themes, Parts I & II.* New York: Theatre Communications Group.

22. Monette P. 1998. *Borrowed Time: An AIDS Memoir.* New York: Harcourt, Brace.

23. Fee E. 2006. The AIDS Memorial Quilt. *American Journal of Public Health* 96(6):979.

TWO: How the Visual Arts Capture the Complexity of Addiction

1. Henningfield, Santora, Bickel, 2007.

Epilogue

1. Henningfield, Santora, Bickel, 2007.

2. Marlatt G. 1980. A cognitive-behavioral model of the relapse process. In NA Krasnegor (Ed.), *Behavioral Analysis and Treatment of Substance Abuse.* Rockville, MD: National Institute on Drug Abuse. Brigham J, Henningfield JE, Stitzer ML. 1990–1991. Smoking relapse: a review. *International Journal of the Addictions* 25(9A–10A):1239–1255. Epstein DH, Willner-Reid J, Vahabzadeh M, Mezghanni M, Lin J-L, Preston KL. 2009. Real-time electronic diary reports of cue exposure and mood in the hours before cocaine and heroin craving and use. *Archives of General Psychiatry* 66(1):88–94.

3. Marlatt G, Gordon JR (Eds.).1985. *Relapse Prevention: Maintenance Strategies in the Treatment of Addictive Behaviors.* New York: Guilford Press.

INDEX OF CONTRIBUTING ARTISTS

Index of Contributing Artists